Live Longer
Live Healthier

The Power of Pycnogenol

Live Longer Live Healthier

The Power of Pycnogenol

The Practical Handbook of Antioxidants

by

Hasnain Walji, Ph.D.

Hohm Press, Prescott, AZ

All Rights Reserved

Hohm Press

PO Box 2501

Prescott, AZ 86302

520-778-9189

Typesetting and layout: AV Communications, Mesa, AZ

Cover: Kim Johansen, Black Dog Design

Library of Congress Cataloguing-in-Publication-Data:
Walji, Hasnain.
    Live longer live healthier : the practical handbook of
antioxidants : the power of pycnogenol / Hasnain Walji.
        p. cm.
    Includes bibliographical references and index.
    ISBN: 0-934252-63-7
    1. Bioflavanoids—Physiological effect. 2. Antioxidants
I. Title.
QP772.B5W35 1996   96-2611
                                             CIP

Disclaimer: Any information in this book is not intended
to be a replacement for medical advice. Any person with
a condition requiring medical attention should consult a
qualified health professional. Further, the author and
publisher claim no endorsement by the manufacturers of
Pycnogenol® (Horphag Research) for the material contained in this book.

Dedication

To the seekers of optimum health and those who help them find it; and to all those teachers who help us all see and search even beyond.

Other books by Hasnain Walji, Ph.D.

The Vitamin Guide: Essential Nutrients for Healthy Living. (Dorset, U.K.: *Element Books*, 1992)

Vitamins, Minerals and Dietary Supplements: A Definitive Guide to Healthy Eating. (London: *Hodder Headline Plc.*, 1994)

Asthma and Hayfever: Combining Orthodox and Complementary Approaches. (London: *Hodder Headline Plc.*, 1994)

Alcohol, Smoking and Tranquillisers. (London: *Hodder Headline Plc.*, 1993)

Heart Health: A Self-Help Guide to Combining Orthodox and Complementary Approaches. (London: *Hodder Headline Plc.*, 1993)

Arthritis and Rheumatism: Orthodox and Complementary Approaches. (London: *Hodder Headline Plc.*, 1994)

Skin Conditions: Orthodox and Complementary Approaches. (London: *Hodder Headline Plc.*, 1993)

Headaches and Migraines: Orthodox and Complementary Approaches. (London: *Hodder Headline Plc.*, 1994)

Healthy Eating. (Cleaveland, U.K.: *C.P.R. Publishing*, 1995)

Using Aromatherapy at Home. (Cleaveland, U.K., 1994)

Melatonin. (London: *Thorsons-HarperCollins*, 1995)

Vitamin C. (London: *Thorsons-HarperCollins*, 1995)

Folic Acid. (London: *Thorsons-HarperCollins*, 1996)

Propolis and Other Nutrients from the Hive. (London: *Thorsons-HarperCollins*, 1996)

The Healing Powers of Aromatherapy (Rockwell, CA: *Prima Publishing*, 1996)

Acknowledgements

I would like to express my deep gratitude to David Ponsonby for assisting me with the research for this book.

I must also acknowledge the quiet encouragement and positivity exuded by Regina Sara Ryan, my editor at Hohm Press, which made working on this book so pleasurable.

Last, but not least, I wish to thank my wife, Latifa, for her patience and endurance during my absence from home in the course of research, not to mention her gentle care and concern, which enabled me to complete this book.

Contents

Preface

"Each patient carries his own doctor inside him."

Dr. Albert Schweitzer

It was in the early 70s when, as a journalist working with an international magazine published in London, I was accidentally introduced to what was then fashionably called "alternative medicine." The Medical Editor, an M.D. turned journalist, was on vacation and it fell upon me to fill in for him. Going through his mail I came across an invitation to a seminar on "Holistic Medicine." I decided to check it out.

I entered the seminar room, in this four-hundred-year-old church hall, not too far from Central London, as a cynic. I came out with burning questions about the efficacy of allopathic medicine. About how *wanting* it was in terms of an holistic perspective.

This meeting set me off on a quest—to find more about other healing modalities, initially from a journalistic curiosity, subsequently with a commitment to learn and inform the general public about issues on health and choices in healing methods, many of which remained within the confines of practitioners' clinics or in the ivory towers of medical colleges.

At the time, I learned one of the most basic yet neglected aspects of allopathic healthcare was the lack of effort in educating the patient on his or her ailment. Was it a question of self interest by the allopathic fraternity that its image as a white-coated "god" would be tarnished if the patient became an informed consumer?

The deeper I dug into the concept of healing and holistic medicine, the more apparent it became that what the patient needed first and foremost was education. Not just about the ailment, but something of a more fundamental nature. I began to understand that there was more to healing than going to a doctor, expecting to be healed. Attaining health was not simply a matter saying, "Here doctor! This is my body. It is sick. Go ahead and heal it while I go on with my life with its inherent stress, bad diet, lack of exercise, etc. etc...."

How had this attitude developed, of abandoned responsibility on the patient's part, and godly power on the doctor's part? I wondered. Over the years I have come to realize that it goes back to the reductionist thinking of René Descartes. His dictum, "I think therefore I am," crystallized the concept of separating *res cognitas* (the realm of the mind) and *res extensa* (the realm of matter). His perception of the material world has so permeated our culture that we now commonly view the human body as an elaborate machine made up of assembled parts.

Descartes said, "I consider the human body as a machine. My thought compares the sick man and an ill-made clock with my idea of a healthy man and a well-made clock." This legacy of reductionism has guided and molded the basis of modern medicine up to the present time.

"It is easy for patients to believe that forces outside themselves are responsible for their illness, but as long as they remain entrenched in that belief system, then the solution to cancer and heart disease and degenerative disorders is not going to be forthcoming. You can only bypass the coronary artery so many times; it keeps getting blocked because the source of illness is within," observes Deepak Chopra, author of the mega-best-seller, *Quantum Healing.*

The culture of dependency spawned by modern medical intervention (of curing the sick parts of the body) has conditioned patients to lose faith in their own ability to heal themselves. They have come to rely on medication as a form of reassurance and to believe that the prescription will "cure."

To make matters worse, modern medicine, preoccupied with measurements, statistical models and double-blind crossover studies fails to take into account the person as a whole and appears to preclude the human potential for self-healing. The mind-body relationship has been ignored in healing. Whatever the disease, unless we accept that this mind-body relationship *does* exist it is not possible to achieve true healing/true health and well being.

A good example of the interaction of mind and body is the human immune system; maintenance of health is a matter of keeping the immune system working at its optimum. Since the immune system is indispensable for defense against disease-causing substances, it is all the more important to keep it in pristine condition. However, stress, environmental pollution and emotional problems work to undermine the strength of the immune system. Aging, inflammation and improper functioning of the circulatory and nervous systems often result from the immune system being of "out of joint." This happens when the immune system is invaded by free radicals—toxic by-products of the body's natural metabolic processes that cause oxidative damage to cells and tissues. Over sixty diseases and conditions, including those generally considered by modern medicine to simply be the consequences of aging (like stiff joints, wrinkled skin, arthritis, and heart disease), are now recognized as having free radicals as their major cause.

Aging is inevitable; a fact of life. How we age, though, is very much up to us and that is why some of us age faster than others. The good news is, however, we have the means of slowing the aging process. Correct nutrition and lifestyle measures from a holistic perspective not only add life to your years, but years to your life!

Current research has focused on nutrients called *antioxidants* that are central to keeping the immune system at its optimum level. Beta Carotene, Vitamins C and E, are all antioxidant nutrients which neutralize free radicals. The irony is, much of this information remains within the confines of research institutes, or is often shrouded with claims and counterclaims by vested commercial interests.

This book, one of fourteen others that I have written on the subject of nutrition and natural healing, seeks to bring out the much needed information on an antioxidant substance which has been proven to be *fifty times* more powerful than vitamin E and *twenty times* more powerful than vitamin C as a free radical scavenger. Dubbed as "the youth nutrient," Pycnogenol, in addition to helping retard the aging process, also helps keep skin in healthy condition and returns flexibility to joints, arteries and other tissue.

But, Pycnogenol or any other nutritional supplement should not be viewed in isolation as a magic bullet. It can only be effective if you wish to attain good health and are willing to work at it from an holistic perspective. The M.D. and his/her drugs, the herbalist and his herbs, the aromatherapist and her essential oils, the acupuncturist and his needles, the osteopath and her manipulation, the chiropractor and his subluxations, and even the anthroposophical doctor with his/her art therapy, eurythmy and hydrotherapy cannot heal.

In order to begin the process of healing you must *want* to achieve health. This means the will to get better must be acknowledged. This is where the mind-body interaction comes into play. A cognizance of this body-mind interaction will result in an integration of the body and the mind in the process of achieving wellness. That is what healing is all about.

Having studied many age-old and traditional healing disciplines, based on different world views and cosmological principles, I have noticed that they all have a common thread: they deal with illness by considering the human in the context of his/her relationship with the cosmos.

The Yogic view is that the human body is composed of three different manifestations, namely the physical body (composed of flesh, blood and bone), the subtle body (containing the life force, *Prana*) and the spiritual body (which encompasses universal wisdom).

To the Hawaiians, health means energy. Good health is a state of *ehuehu* (abundant energy) and poor health is *pake* (weakness). Illness is caused by tension (*mai*) and healing is equated to the restoration of energy (*lapau*). Health therefore is "a state of harmonious energy."

According to Ibn Sina, "Muslim physicians consider man as a psychosomatic unity endowed with a self-directed, purposeful *rooh* or vital force."

The American Indians consider that Earth Mother is a living organism, and that all creations on this Earth share a life force; all are part of a harmonious whole. Illness occurs when this balance is upset. The purpose of healing ceremonies, then, is to restore both personal and universal harmony.

Tai chi is the Chinese way of increasing the energy flow in the body and strengthening the body's resistance to ward off disease. *Tai chi* is thought to stimulate the kidney meridian (seen as the life force energy) and to maintain vitality of mind, body and spirit.

Rudolph Steiner, the founder of anthroposophy, sought to go beyond the idea of healing the body. His acute perception led him to explore the spiritual side of existence which led to an understanding of the ways of stimulating the natural healing forces in the person. Healing was a matter of considering the interrelation between the four aspects of the human being (physical body, etheric body, astral body and the ego) and treating them as a whole.

The similarities are striking! Call it by any name— *prana, rooh, chi,* life force, *ehuehu,* etheric energy—we all have it in us. It's up to the "doctor inside," to borrow Albert Schweitzer's phrase, to harness this healing force within us and so to achieve that state of balance among body, mind and spirit.

Hasnain Walji
January 1996

Live Longer
Live Healthier

The Power of Pycnogenol

Chapter 1

What is Pycnogenol?

PYCNOGENOL (pick-nah-geh-nol), a classic example of a plant or herbal medicine derived from the knowledge of indigenous people, was originally extracted from pine bark, although grape seeds now occupy a significant segment of the raw material.

Pycnogenol consists primarily of a special blend of bioflavonoids, termed "proanthocyanidins." Curiously, these proanthocyanidins, in the artificial form of an isolated extract, play a unique role independent of any vitamin C supplementation; but they also potentiate the action of vitamin C when taken in combination with it. Pycnogenol alone or vitamin C alone are not as effective as the two together!

At one time, as a bioflavonoid, Pycnogenol would have enjoyed the status of being a vitamin—"Vitamin P." There are a number of advantages inherent in this vitamin classification. Some researchers believe that, in the "light" of recent research, a reexamination of the status of bioflavonoids as a vitamin in their own right is in order. There is considerable support for the restoration of its lost classification. The growing interest in natural products has already led to a "catch-phrase" designation of a *"phytamin,"* or the more formal *"phytotherapy."*

Used in Europe for many decades, both as a supplement and on prescription, Pycnogenol has recently been patented in the United States and is now available as a nutritional supplement. As a class of vitamin it would enjoy special status. The issue of herbal medicines, however, would complicate matters, possibly requiring drug status and ultimately removing it from over-the-counter (otc) availability. (Such has been the fate of Melatonin given its recent publicity in both Canada and England—although, of course, Melatonin is a hormone rather than a nutrient and is not derived from plant sources.)

Pycnogenol (in common with vitamins A, C and E) acts independently as an antioxidant to reduce the damage caused by free radicals. Taken along with Vitamin C, Pycnogenol potentiates (acts as a "helper") the numerous biological functions which have been identified for vitamin C—and there are literally hundreds.

History

The history of Pycnogenol, or more accurately a concoction (herbal tea) derived from the pine tree, dates back to the sixteenth century and the discovery of Canada's Gulf of St. Lawrence by the French explorer, Jacques Cartier.

The story goes that the Cartier expedition to Canada during the winter of 1534 was prevented from leaving St. Lawrence by ice in the waterways. As their supplies were diminishing rapidly, they landed in the Quebec peninsula to hunt for food. Proceeding on their voyage, they survived on rations of salted meat and biscuits; they had no fruits or vegetables in their diet. By December 1534 they were struck down with scurvy (now recognized as a vitamin C deficiency disease) losing twenty-five of the one-hundred ten men in the crew. Many more men were rapidly succumbing to the dreaded disease, while the local inhabitants seemed to remain healthy, unperturbed by such ravages of winter. Finally, the remaining crew were saved by these local Indians who told them about a tea made from the bark and needles of a local maritime pine, and showed them how to brew it. This pine was described by Cartier as the Anneda tree, with evergreen leaves and an easy-to-remove bark. We now know that the needles contained small amounts of Vitamin C and the bark contained compounds called flavonols.

One can only presume that some innate intelligence aided the indigenous peoples of Canada in identifying this Vitamin C source in the first place. The same innate intelligence seems to have guided the natives in their use of animal food—even when there was an abundant supply of game, the local inhabitants carefully utilized it. The native hunters knew to eat the adrenal glands of their prey. (We now know that animals must produce their own vitamin C, and that it is stored in their adrenal glands.) Europeans, on the other hand, when faced with an abundant food supply tended to eat only the same choice cuts, like venison steak from deer, or tongue from the buffalo.

The first recorded beneficiaries of what has become known as "Pycnogenol" were the sailors and explorers of the Cartier expedition. It is ironic, however, that scurvy continued to be a major killer of sailors for several centuries after Cartier's experience. The link between scurvy and vitamin C remained "undiscovered" for several centuries, gaining credence again only after the successful voyages of Captain James Cook who circumnavigated the world in the late eighteenth century without losing a man to scurvy. Part of his armamentarium, along with citrus fruits, was spruce beer! *= equipment, armory 2 equipments and methods used in medicine*

(Incidentally, most "recruits" were acquired by the so-called "Press Gangs," whereby the slightly inebriated customers of public houses near the docks would be bumped on the head, only to wake up on board one of His Majesty's ships of the line. Discipline was harsh. Obedience and victory might be rewarded with rum and beer. Any hesitation would *earn* the infamous "Cat O' Nine Tails," a whip with nine sections.)

Spruce beer: a beverage flavored with with spruce esp-one made from spruce twigs and leaves then boiled together with molasses and fermented with yeast r and sugar

3

The first scientific discovery of this link between Vitamin C and scurvy was made by the Scottish physician James Lind in 1753. In those days, when sailors set out to sea their rations consisted of salted beef, biscuits and water. Frequently the men would develop weakness, swollen and bleeding gums; their teeth would drop out, joints would swell, old wounds would reopen. Eventually, many sailors died. Scurvy (for this is what the disease was) became the major cause of death at sea. Lind maintained that the cure for this disease was lime juice and, following his recommendations, sailors began to take provisions of limes with them on their long voyages.

In 1795, the British Navy finally issued general orders to provide lime juice (as well as rum) to its sailors: hence the generic term for the English as "Limeys." Sailors of other nations only gained parity by the mid-nineteenth century.

It was as late as the 1930's when this Vitamin C-link was finally established by Hungarian scientist Albert Szent-Gyorgyi. In animal studies, he also discovered that crude extracts from lemon juice were more effective against scurvy than pure vitamin C (or ascorbic acid). Szent-Gyorgyi further found that administering lemon juice was effective in strengthening capillaries, whereas ascorbic acid on its own was ineffective. This led to the isolation of a compound from lemon rind which he called vitamin P (permeability vitamin). Vitamin P was later recognized as one of the bioflavonoids which enhances the benefits of vitamin C. To date, over twenty thousand bioflavonoids have been identified.

It is now understood why Cartier's sailors benefited from pine needles and bark. This herbal tea not only prevented deterioration in the sailors' health (this deterioration which had formerly left them defenseless against the ravages of the disease). But, even if the disease had already taken hold, in the early stages, the tea could achieve a reversal in the condition, effectively healing the sailors' wounds and saving their lives.

4

Almost four hundred years after Cartier's narrow escape, a French scientist by the name of Professor Jacques Masquelier of Bordeaux began investigating the biochemistry of this tea that cured scurvy. He realized that there couldn't be much vitamin C in pine needles and certainly none in the bark. Yet, the Indians had achieved remarkable results, apparently potentiating the meager amounts of vitamin C through these co-factors.

This led Masquelier to isolate the healing bioflavonoid from the pine tree. At first, he believed there was only one compound: leucocyanidin. He coined the word *pycnogenols* to describe this compound. Later, he was able to show that the compound was an entire class of bioflavonoids called proanthocyanidins. In France the term for proanthocyanidins is OPC's.

Masquelier's extract was first patented in 1982, (the manufacturing being done in Switzerland) and he was issued a U.S. patent in 1987.

OPC's have been extracted from pine bark since the early 1950's, when Jacques Masquelier patented the extraction process. In the early 1970's, Prof. Masquelier discovered that the extraction process used for pine bark would also extract OPC's from grape seed (Vitus vinifera). His pioneering work into the antioxidant properties of OPC's from grape seeds soon followed, culminating in a 1987 U.S. patent (#4,698,360), titled: *"Plant Extract with a Proanthocyanidins Content as Therapeutic Agent Having Radical Scavenger Effect and Use Thereof."* He and others then performed extensive analytical, toxicological, pharmacological, and clinical studies using the grape seed extract.

In the 1991 publication, *"Historical Note On OPC,"* Professor Masquelier states, "OPC from grape pips [seeds] has an advantage over OPC from pine bark. OPC from grape pips contains the gallic esters of proanthocyanidins (in particular: B 2 – 3' – O – gallate). These proanthocyanidin-esters have been recently described as the most active substances in the battle against free radicals."

Ecologically, grape seed is also a preferred source of Pycnogenols, as only the fruit is harvested. In contrast, the bark of the Maritime pine is used for the pine bark extract. (The trees are not harvested solely for their bark and only a small fraction of the bark is diverted from the main lumber industry of the region for Pycnogenol production. For the record, it takes about one ton of pine bark to produce five pounds of Pycnogenol.) The grape seed extract is also less expensive.

Dr. Masquelier now uses the term OPC-85 for pine bark extract and OPC–85+ for grape seed extract. The pine bark and grape seed extracts can both be produced under Prof. Masquelier's patented process.

Masquelier was associated with the Swiss Company, Horphag, from 1951 until 1991. The term "Pycnogenol" was claimed by Horphag Research and is a registered trademark for their products sold in the United States.

At first, due to exclusivity arrangements with the pharmaceutical company marketing the grape seed extract in France as a pharmaceutical product, only the pine bark extract was available for the U.S. market. The pine bark extract is also more expensive, which may also have appealed to the multi-level marketing firms responsible for its initial distribution.

The grape seed extract became available within the United States in 1992 and, in spite of its lower price, is reputed to provide the higher quality proanthocyanidins; hence its inclusion in "professional" lines.

Consumer products now tend to be a blend of both sources (pine bark and grape seed). Various claims and counter-claims are made by the vested interest groups so that it is difficult to generalize about the true superiority enjoyed by any one version of the product.

Chapter 2

Basic Chemistry

PROANTHOCYANIDINS (PAC's) are composed of polyphenols, or Oligomeric Proanthocyanadin Complexes (OPC's) which are defined by the exclusive property of producing a red pigment (anthocyanidin), hence the efficacy of red grapes and red wine. There are, in fact, several procyanidins: oligomeric and monomeric. About 85% of the compounds of Pycnogenol have been identified as procyanidins. Of these, about 60% are oligomeric procyanidins (OPC's): dimers, trimers and tetramers of catechin and epicatechin; 20% are oligomers and phenolic acids such as gallic acid.

Chemically, therefore, Pycnogenol appears to be complex, which is an accurate reflection of its composition. It is not a simple bioflavonoid. The extract is made with water, hence all of these components are water soluble. However, their chemical make-up is diverse. Just because a component is present in minuscule quantities should not detract from its contribution to the overall efficacy of the total package.

Briefly, for those whose curiosity has been aroused and who may not possess an advanced chemistry book, the essential differences between the classifications mentioned is outlined next.

A monomer is a single molecule. A dimer is formed by two identical molecules, like hydrogen's contribution to

7

water (H_2O). An oligomer is a larger compound of molecules and a polymer is a very large compound. In everyday life we encounter quite a few polymers. Most homeowners will be familiar with polyurethane and polystyrene in the form of paint and foam, respectively. The advantages are dependent upon the inherent rigidity of large molecules.

For those who like a more tangible, nutritional, or dietary reference point, these plant extracts may simply be regarded as esters of bioflavonols. On a more mundane level, another close relative, with a long history of consumption, especially in Japan, is green tea.

Bioflavonoids

Bioflavonoids and carotenoids provide the variation of colors in the vegetable kingdom. Chlorophyll provides the green which is the central component of a plant's energy system; bioflavonoids contribute blues, purples, emerald green and some reds; carotenoids provide the yellow-orange-red hues (like carrots). They are concentrated in the skins and seeds. Flavonoids function to screen plants from light.

It has long been known that consuming whole fruits and vegetables provided an enhanced nutrition over and above even mega-dosage supplementation with vitamin C. The bioflavonoids have even been added to some vitamin C preparations in order to more closely approximate the natural bounty of raw, fresh fruits and vegetables. Oranges may contain over forty flavonoids, while there are thousands overall.

Production

In brief, the raw material (pine bark or grape seeds) is processed to exclude waste material and the OPC's are ultimately extracted with water, so that its constituents are water soluble. This is usually touted to be a strong-point, in that Pycnogenol will be easily assimilated by the body...it is *bioavailable*.

This also means that it will only remain in the body temporarily and must be replaced on a daily basis in order to maintain saturation levels.

However, Dr. Marc S. Micozzi has set out his opposing viewpoint. Dr. Micozzi is a medical anthropologist, among other things (nutritionist, oncologist, pathologist), which leads him to conclude that humans have been herbivorous throughout their existence, and should therefore continue to eat plant foods, whole. As bioflavonoids are not very water-soluble, they do not find their way into juice very well, so we must devour the whole fruit or vegetable. Micozzi does not believe that supplements offer the same range of nutrients as the raw, whole version.

Most supplement manufacturers, of course, could not deny Micozzi's claim but would emphasize the benefit of a concentrated source. After all, how many of us could or would consume, every day, the several pounds of fruits and vegetables necessary to get the active ingredients which are purportedly contained within a few tablets?

Anyone wishing to delve deeper into the chemistry and pharmacology of Pycnogenol can look up the pertinent references. (See Abstracts and References, pp. 73-85.) It is beyond the scope of our present work to discuss them all here. You don't need to understand the biochemistry or different chemical structures in order to appreciate Pycnogenol.

what is a drug anyway?
a substance intended to be used for diagnosis,
cure, mitigation, treatment or prevention
for a desease 2 a substance other than
food intended to affect the structure
or function of the body.

Chapter 3
(3) an illegal substance as narcotics
that causes an addiction

Is Pycnogenol a Drug? *crab or*
habituation or
a marked change in consciousness

IN SOME countries, like France and Germany, certain Pycnogenol products have been designated as "drugs" in order to achieve reimbursable status.

In the United States, the costly process to achieve "drug" status boosts the desirability of retaining a food classification/(herbal) product with no direct health claims. This category has been coming under attack from certain quarters, as the medical establishment and pharmaceutical industry seek to gain control of the health food and nutritional supplement industries.

Innocently, the indigenous people of Canada used an herbal product—bark and needles—to concoct a tea to ward off winter diseases (like scurvy). Pycnogenol is refined from this material, ending up as a purified *nutrient* closely related to vitamin C and bioflavonoids. And, as was mentioned in Chapter 1, bioflavonoids even had the distinction of being a vitamin temporarily ("vitamin P"). Left simply as a nutritional supplement, without any direct prescription for diseases, the nutrient classification for Pycnogenol is in order. No expensive trials need to be undertaken within the United States under the supervision of the FDA (Food and Drug Administration).

According to researchers, Uchida and Edamastu, with the Department of Pharmacy at Nagasaki University School of Medicine in Japan, Pycnogenol has been found to possess twenty times the antioxidant capacity of vitamin C, and to be fifty times more powerful than vitamin E. They used a standard *in vitro* (in a glass dish) chemistry test on free radicals and measured the concentration of the bioflavonoids being tested (Pycnogenol, vitamin C and vitamin E) to inhibit the free radicals by 50%:

"Making use of Electron Spin Resonance" analysis... we found that these bioflavonoids had a potent scavenging action toward active oxygen free radicals...The bioflavonoids...warrant further study as a promising alternative in the prevention and therapy of several diseases attributed to reactions of oxygen free radicals." ("Condensed Tannins Scavenge Active Oxygen Radicals." *Medical Science Research.* [1980]; 15: 831–2.)

Supporting work has been conducted by French researchers in Dijon.

Flavonoids are natural antioxidants. Flavonoids have been evaluated in the treatment of several human diseases, including cancer. Some studies found that flavonoids had a protective effect against carcinogens, not only at a cellular or enzymatic level, but also by reducing their bioavailability. Animal data suggests that polyphenols could hinder the uptake of some xenobiotics from the gastrointestinal tract. The results of this study with quercetin, ellagic acid and chlorogenic acid show their benefit by the reduction of the bioavailability of carcinogens. (Stavric, B., and T.I Matula. "Flavonoids in Foods: Their Significance For Nutrition and Health." *Lipid Soluble Antioxidants: Biochemistry and Clinical Applications.* [1992]; 274–294.)

Failure to take Pycnogenol has not been proven to result in a specific disease process—hence it is not recognized as a true vitamin. In other words, there is no Pycnogenol-deficiency state! However, there is no shortage of publications chock-full of reports about the benefits to be gained from supplementing with Pycnogenol. For the moment, you must judge for yourself.

This book will detail available evidence and claims regarding the supplementation of the diet with Pycnogenol, but no such claims can accompany the product itself. To do so would constitute a claim for Pycnogenol to be considered as a drug; and that would have to be substantiated to the satisfaction of the FDA. This is another reason why so many of the trials and claims derive from Europe whereas any American experiences quoted will fall into the "anecdotal" category, i.e. subjective, personal accounts not subjected to scientific inquiry, clinical trials and (medical) peer review.

In order to understand the way Pycnogenol can be beneficial, it is important to look at the way the body fights disease. The well-known role of vitamin C also serves as a benchmark, since Pycnogenol not only contributes its own antioxidant activity, but additionally boosts the action of vitamin C.

benchmark: a mark on a permanent object indicating elevation and serving as a reference from which measurements in topographical surveys and tidal observation

2 something that is taken as a standard by which others can be measured or judged.

3 a basis for evaluation.

*Desease = the breakdown of the body's
natural functions*

*antioxidants = enzymes that act
as protectors against
body damages
(skin cancer, wrinkles ~
and modern life diet.
and from "free Radicals" as
herbicides, pesticides, pollution,
Sun light, tabaco smoke, even exercise*

Chapter 4

Disease Fighter

MOST of us learn how the pristine appearance of our shiny new bike (or car, or house) seldom lasts very long, especially if we scratch it or leave it out in the sun and weather. We learn that nature is relentless. We must toil laboriously with polishes and paints to fight a losing battle, victorious if we succeed in extending the lifespan of our bike or car or house by a few years.

Our bodies are much the same. Look at the ravages of exposing our skin to the great outdoors: skin cancer and wrinkles. Naturally, the body has a fail-safe mechanism to protect us against such damage, but these resources (enzymes called antioxidants) tend to be in short supply with our modern diet, whereas the "enemy" (free radicals) is everywhere. The free radicals generated by herbicides, pesticides, pollution, sunlight, tobacco smoke, even exercise etc., are more powerful and numerous than ever before.

The Role of Nutrition in Health

Both orthodox and alternative health practitioners will tell you that underlying all disease is the breakdown of the body's natural functions. Poor nutrition is one of the primary causes of such a breakdown.

*our enemy = (free radicals) = herbicides
Pesticides
Pollution
Sun light
Tabaco Smoke, Exercise*

13

Hippocrates, the Father of Medicine, recognized this two thousand years ago. Sadly, his words, "Let food be your medicine, and your medicine be your food," seem to have been lost to the modern era.

Our current sophisticated knowledge of the disease process has led to the production of specific drugs to counteract symptoms... if only for short-term benefit. They are strictly palliative! Such drugs may help to relieve the symptoms but they do not prevent them from recurring. A return to basics, to food as medicine, is what is really needed.

The body, through its immune system, has an amazing capacity to deal with the viruses, bacteria and other organisms that are an integral part of our lives. Yet, we are now less able to fight disease. The understanding is only just emerging that changes in lifestyle and eating habits during the last one hundred years have heaped an untold burden on our bodies.

It used to be said that, "You are what you eat." Now, our food is grown with artificial fertilizers, and subjected to refining and processing so that few nutrients remain. Nonetheless, our need for these nutrients has increased tremendously. Hence, it is now becoming popular to say that, "You are what you assimilate."

In present day America, most people suffer from a new form of *malnutrition*, they are obese (one-third of the population is overweight by most estimates) from too many calories but still undernourished! Lack of nutrients weakens the body's various systems, including the immune system, and impairs its function. To understand this is to understand the role of nutrition in the prevention of disease.

Chapter 5

The Immune System

OUR IMMUNE SYSTEM is the body's main line of defense against both minor and major illnesses. The first line of defense against these assailants is the skin, which is our largest organ. The large molecules it contains, as well as the mucous membranes (and their associated fluids) present in the body's openings, have immunological properties and are also naturally acidic.

Furthermore, the outer skin as well as the membranes lining the digestive system, play host to millions of *friendly* germs that fend off *harmful* ones.

If an attacking micro-organism makes it past the first barrier, it next encounters the phagocytes. These are white blood cells which eat and destroy foreign substances. There are two sorts of phagocyte—the macrophages and the microphages.

As their name suggests, *macrophages* are large cells that surround and eat up dead tissue and cells. These special cells are found in the regional lymph nodes (we are all painfully aware of how swollen these become during an infection; neck, armpit, groin being key areas).

If the macrophages cannot deal with the enemy, they call for reinforcements: microphages. These destroy bacteria. As soon as the immune system encounters a germ or a bug that it perceives as foreign, certain cells in the body fight the organism to get rid of it.

Visualize an army, with its ranks of generals down to the lowest foot soldier, and you will be able to imagine how the immune system works.

Phagocytes provide interim protection until the immune system has marshalled all its forces and is ready to go into operation. Its army comprises specialist organs and cells; the *major* gland is the thymus.

First, there are the *leukocytes*. These are white blood cells that scavenge the enemy. There are five types of leukocyte—each with a different part to play. The most plentiful of these are the *neutrophils*, whose job it is to "eat up" the enemy cells which are the first to reach the site of infection. *Eosinophils* fight allergies and infections from parasites. They are very active in the later stages of an infection, and increase during the healing stages of an inflammation.

Basophils are involved in the battle against blood diseases and some abnormalities of the bone marrow and spinal cord. They are released in chronic inflammation and the healing stages.

Lymphocytes are the main fighting forces in the leukocyte army. They are formed in the lymph nodes and help to combat viral infections.

Last, there are the *monocytes*, which fight chronic infection by helping to rid the body of damaged and dead cells. They also prepare body tissue for healing.

It is the lymphocytes that the macrophages call on if they are overwhelmed by the enemy. There are two divisions of lymphocytes—the T-cells and the B-cells. The T-cells are highly specialized cells that engage in what may be called "hand-to-hand" combat with the invader; T-cells have a regulatory function. They fight fungi, viruses, some bacteria, tumors and transplanted cells.

There are helper T-cells, suppressor T-cells and cyto-toxic T-cells. The helper T-cells secrete a substance called interleukin-2, and this increases the activity of the other T-cells. Usually, several of these immune system substances are included in any investigation into cancer and AIDS.

B-cells are manufactured in the bone marrow and pass through an area in the intestines. B-lymphocytes secrete highly effective, defensive proteins called antibodies. They are vital for defending the body against pus-producing bacteria. B-cells break down into plasma cells, which manufacture protein molecules called antibodies, and memory cells. The foreign substances that stimulate the production of antibodies are called antigens.

Antibodies also have another name: *immunoglobulins*, because they are found in the globulin part of blood proteins. There are five types of immunoglobulin. (Immunoglobulin G) IgG is the most important of these. It can squeeze between cells and enter tissue. It neutralizes micro-organisms.

IgA provides immunity for the body's orifices and is present in breastmilk (as is IgG).

IgM is the largest of the antibodies and remains in the blood where it kills bacteria.

IgD is found almost only in the cell membranes and controls their behavior.

IgE is responsible for releasing histamines into the blood.

Certain glands and organs are also components of the immune system and they work together with the army of cells.

Red bone marrow produces the red blood cells and is the "training ground" for the lymphocytes. It also makes *granulocytes*, *monocytes* and *platelets* for the bloodclotting process.

The *thymus* gland is where the lymphocytes actually originate and it stimulates the development of those cells into plasma cells. Its main function seems to be in the manufacture and export of immunologically competent T-cells to other parts of the body, such as the spleen and the lymph nodes.

The *lymphatic* system is involved in the collection, filtration and redirection of lymph into the bloodstream and back to the heart. Lymph is the fluid that leaks from the blood through the walls of the tiny blood vessels called capillaries. This fluid bathes the body cells and tissues and provides nourishment in the form of oxygen. The nodes that do the filtering are situated throughout the body. They are the most important source of antibodies. Lymph nodes filter bacteria from the lymph stream to prevent the spread of infection.

The spleen is involved in blood formation, storage and filtration.

The intestinal walls contain aggregated lymphatic nodules named after the anatomist, Peyer: *"Peyers' Patches,"* which provide a defense mechanism against intestinal invaders. *Tonsils* act as a filter, protecting against bacteria. The *adenoids* and the *appendix* have similar functions.

Another part of the immune system is found in the thymus gland (the "general" in this army). When the system is activated by a foreign organism this is known as the *adaptive response*. However, the system, having once encountered a particular invader, is able to "remember" the organism and, as soon as it is encountered again, mobilizes its forces much more efficiently.

If there is a breakdown in any of the components of the immune system, the body's ability to fight disease is severely impaired. The result is that many of us live with recurring health problems—colds, flu, chronic fatigue and other diseases including hay fever and asthma.

If the system is working well, then we either do not become ill or, if we do, we are able to recover quickly.

Acquired Immunity

Vaccination is a good illustration of the workings of the immune system. A small amount of treated or dead organism is introduced into the body by injecting a vaccine. As the organism is already treated or dead, there is no danger of acquiring the disease. However, as soon as the body's defense force encounters the foreign organism, the defense force is put on red alert—fights the invader and makes antibodies to it. The body will also remember how to get rid of this organism should it meet a similar one in the future. So, if you were again to become infected with an active, live organism of the same kind, say of smallpox or cholera, your immune system would be able to respond to it before the foreign organism had a chance to cause disease.

All immunity information is stored in the thymus gland, the body's "computer." It instructs the body's defense force when to commence attack and, equally, when not to attack in the case of harmless foreign organisms.

Sometimes the immune system malfunctions or is seriously weakened, with potentially grave consequences. One example of a malfunction of a relatively minor nature is that which results in hay fever. In this instance the immune system over-reacts to a harmless substance such as pollen. The system releases a substance called histamine into the bloodstream in an effort to wash away the intruder. A more serious form of malfunction is when the immune system starts attacking the body's own cells, as happens with rheumatoid arthritis. The most infamous example of an auto-immune disorder is, of course, **Acquired-Immune-Deficiency-Syndrome**, i.e. AIDS.

The immune system may also break down or become weakened as a result of what is termed "toxic overload." This overload is attributable to the many pollutants with which we are assailed and which our bodies have never before encountered. Toxic materials which cannot be broken down by the body and excreted are stored in our body fats, the liver, bones and even the brain. Stress, with the consequent overproduction of adrenaline, can also contribute to a weakened immune system. A nutritionally inadequate diet only makes the situation worse.

People whose immune systems are not "up to scratch" (no pun intended) will find themselves coming down with one cold after another. They will suffer from chronic fatigue and health problems. Ultimately they may succumb to more damaging diseases—for example, cancer.

Everyone's body produces cancer cells, hundreds of them on a daily basis, but for most people the immune systems take care of them. When the immune system is suppressed, these cells get out of control and proliferate, becoming more difficult to control, by any means.

As long as the immune system is healthy it can fend off the onslaught of disease but it can be compromised by poor diet, environmental pollution, stress and even the natural process of aging, with serious consequences.

You can see how important it is to keep the immune system in a state of balance. However, the problem for the immune system in this late twentieth century is that while the human body is remarkably adaptable in its quest for survival, it needs time to change.

Unfortunately, the pace of change in the environment has overtaken the body's natural ability to offer a timely response. The immune system is overworked and does not always know how to respond to the array of new enemies that confront it. Environmental pollution, the depletion of the ozone layer, pesticides and CFCs have all contributed in upsetting our finely tuned immune system.

Furthermore, if the system cannot eliminate and detoxify a foreign organism, the body has to store it somewhere. The liver, bones, and even the brain become the storehouses for this sometimes dangerous waste. The effects of these toxins, together with the imbalance of nutrients in our food increases our vulnerability to disease.

Oxygen—The Main Culprit!

Something not good may be beneficial or vis eversa

Oxygen is necessary to sustain life but, paradoxically, it can also become the chief culprit. All living things that use oxygen produce free radicals. Free radicals are the cause of rusting iron, hardened rubber and wrinkled skin. When cells use oxygen, they inevitably produce a small proportion of unstable molecules that lack an electron (molecules are stable only when they are electronically even). These unstable oxygen molecules are free radicals.

Created every minute we are alive, free radicals are largely held in check by the body's own army of antioxidants, and as long as they are kept under control we remain healthy. However, if we begin to make more free radicals than we need (and they do serve a useful function), there is a risk of damage to the immune system and of developing chronic diseases.

Unchecked free radicals are thought to be the major cause of mutations and cancers, memory loss and senility, autoimmune diseases, aging and wrinkles.

To help our understanding, visualize the errant behavior of a free radical as a lonely spark of electricity dashing around looking to bind with a companion electron, thereby neutralizing the original antagonist but, at the same time, creating another "orphan" radical. So the hunt proceeds unabated, like musical chairs, as lone radicals seek partners, breaking up existing pairs in the process.

According to medical researcher Dr. Parris Kidd: "Free radical chain reactions can be lethal to cells and tissues.

21

The lipid (fatty) membranes, which are key workbenches for the cell, are particularly susceptible. Free radicals can also damage the enzymes that are necessary for the more than one hundred thousand reactions of metabolism. Given the chance, free radicals will damage genes, punch holes in cells, break down tissues, and, as a consequence, destroy the functions of entire organs. Exposure to free radicals over a long period is likely to cause degenerative...diseases, to trigger autoimmune diseases...and to accelerate aging." (*The Vitamin Connection*, July/August 1988, p. 16).

A Weakened Immune System

As we have seen before, free radicals have to take much of the blame for a weakened immune system. Most of us are in a state of deficit expenditure, or disease. We are, literally, over-run by free radicals. Many of the normal activities of our cells result in the production of free radicals. Most of them are the by-product of the process of making energy from oxygen. They have been described as "an unavoidable genetic flaw of this process." Normally, our bodies can protect themselves from free radicals going out of control and attacking the body, by drawing on our resources of antioxidants.

Arteries can become clogged up, the cells in artery walls (particularly susceptible as they are made up of polyunsaturated fats that can go rancid through being oxidized by free radicals) may die—causing heart disease. The chances of contracting cancer are increased through damaged DNA. Mutations, memory loss, senility and wrinkles can all be attributable to free radical attack.

Environmental Factors That Add to the Free Radical Burden

Not only must our bodies cope with the free radicals naturally occurring within; they must also try to handle novel, outside factors which increase free radical production still more by depleting the antioxidants in body tissues. Such factors include:

- excessive exposure to X-rays
- radioactive contamination
- pesticides, industrial solvents, and CFCs
- cigarette smoke
- radiation
- burns, excessive heat or cold
- surgery
- infection, e.g. by viruses & bacteria, pesticide residues, household chemicals
- certain drugs
- nitrites, nitrates and other food additives

Protection From Free Radicals

Protection from free radicals comes from antioxidants. An antioxidant is a substance that can protect foods from oxidation (going rancid)—especially fats and oils. It does this by preventing oxygen from combining with other substances and damaging cells.

The nutrients that are commonly thought of as our first line of defense against free radical attack are vitamins A (beta carotene), C and E; and minerals: zinc and selenium. (Some amino acids also have a part to play in fighting excess free radicals but most amino acids—the so-called *non-essential* can be produced by the body).

Recent research has introduced two new players into the antioxidant mix: melatonin, a hormone principally secreted by the pineal gland; and, of course, the complex that has come to be known as Pycnogenol.

Vitamins and minerals cannot be produced by the body itself and must come from the diet, demonstrating how important the relationship is between sound nutrition and a healthy immune system.

Chapter 6

Protective Nutrients

THE STATEMENT that "we are overfed but undernourished" makes sense once we understand why, despite having all the food we need, we still remain short of essential nutrients.

Our diets abound in proteins, carbohydrates and fats. These are called *macronutrients* and form the bulk of the food we eat. Vitamins and minerals, although essential, are only required in minute quantities (*micronutrients*). Macronutrients provide energy. Micronutrients (which neither contain calories nor provide energy themselves) allow energy to be released. Vitamins and minerals, in fact, are a part of the structure of enzymes (organic catalysts that facilitate the complex biological processes). Disease can develop if these micronutrients are consistently missing from our daily diet.

Micronutrients are delicate and can easily be destroyed or depleted by a whole host of factors. Modern farming methods have depleted the minerals in soil. The use of pesticides together with food processing technology have further reduced the levels of these essential nutrients in our food

A deficiency of certain nutrients means that other nutrients cannot be fully absorbed and the digestive functions are disturbed.

As far as asthma and hay fever are concerned, the body needs higher than normal levels of certain nutrients to counter the effects of inflammation and the overreaction of the immune system.

As previously mentioned, certain vitamins and minerals also function as antioxidants. By eating whole foods that are rich in these micronutrients we can increase our intake of these antioxidants. The World Health Organization (WHO) has recently recommended a daily intake of 400 g (approximately 1 lb.) of fruit and vegetables (to include beans and pulses) to keep us healthy. However, this is not always possible or practical, and vitamin supplements can help "bridge the gap."

Antioxidants Play a Key Role

The absence of adequate levels of antioxidants seems to play a key role in the development of certain neurodegenerative diseases, as well as cancer and heart disease. Logically, the longer such deficiencies have existed, the more likely a disease state will develop. Hence, many diseases are commonly considered to be the inevitable consequence of aging (although not every aged person, of course, suffers from them). The explanation may be that it is not the number of years someone has lived that is important, but rather a cumulative effect of the imbalance between the amount of antioxidant deficiency relative to free radical exposure.

The first principal then is that antioxidants can prevent or delay the onset of degenerative diseases. They also seem to be capable of reducing the severity of a pre-existing condition.

Antioxidants also appear to be capable of conferring some degree of resistance to, or immunity against, the invasion of disease organisms, whether bacterial, viral or parasitic.

It may well be that this strengthened immunity is, at least partially, derived from the enhanced quality of rest and sleep obtained by some people through the use of melatonin supplements. The well-rested body is better able to repair itself and face new attacks.

We can reduce our exposure to free radicals by staying out of the sun, wearing sunscreens, getting proper rest and selecting a diet that can provide us with a high level of antioxidant nutrients.

In the context of our frenetic lifestyles, however, it may be more convenient to boost our defenses by supplementation with antioxidants, like Pycnogenol™. Linus Pauling convinced most of us that vitamin C is a powerful antioxidant. Professor Masquelier reports that Pycnogenol is twenty times stronger than vitamin C! Similarly, it is also estimated that Pycnogenol is 50 times more effective than vitamin E.

So, while Pycnogenol may be more powerful than vitamins C and E with respect to some actions, it does not mean that vitamins C and E may be dispensed with altogether in the overpowering presence of Pycnogenol.

Many scientists and physicians now adamantly recommend supplementing our diet, in addition to raising our intake of fruits and vegetables—the natural sources of the vitamins, minerals and bioflavonoids such as Pycnogenol which neutralize free radicals. Let us now look at some of the other protective nutrients that help.

Antioxidant Nutrients

Vitamin A and beta carotene

The mucous membranes in our eyes, ears, nose, throat and lungs all require vitamin A to maintain their stability. Allergens can be kept at bay if the membranes are healthy.

The first fat-soluble vitamin ever to be identified, vitamin A is the general name for a group of substances which include retinol, retinal and the carotenoids. The active forms of vitamin A are found in animal tissue. The carotenoids need bile and fats to be present in the intestines in order to be absorbed. Although this vitamin is stable in light and heat, it is destroyed by the sun's ultraviolet rays and by oxidation, hence the need for vitamin E to be present as well since it sacrifices itself to protect vitamin A.

Beta carotene, derived from vegetable sources, is sometimes referred to as provitamin A. It is found in the yellow pigment present in many fruits and vegetables. Except for diabetics, the human body can readily convert beta carotene into Vitamin A. Beta carotene is thought to be a free radical quencher and so can protect delicate cells from the danger of oxidation.

Vitamin A is found in eggs, milk, lamb's liver, halibut liver oil, cod liver oil, dairy products, pig's kidney, carrots, beef, mackerel and canned sardines. You will find beta carotene in spinach, carrots, kale, broccoli, peaches, apricots— the orange and green vegetables and fruits.

Vitamin B_6

B_6 regulates antibodies and improves the activity of the T- and B-cells in the immune system. In one study patients reported a dramatic decrease in the frequency and severity of wheezing and asthmatic attacks while taking B_6 supplements.

Research undertaken in Mt. Pleasant, Texas, has shown an amazing capacity for vitamin B_6 (pyridoxine) to slow down and even reverse the otherwise inevitable deterioration of vision in the eyes of diabetics ("diabetic retinopathy"). Strengthening the tiny blood vessels in the eye may be associated with antioxidant scavenging of free radicals, and with tissue formation.

Vitamin B_{12}

This vitamin appears to be especially effective in sulphite-sensitive individuals. In one clinical trial weekly injections of 1 mg of B_{12} produced a definite improvement in asthmatic patients.

Vitamin C

This is perhaps the most important nutrient for the immune system. As an antioxidant it aids the immune system; as a natural antihistamine it alleviates the allergic symptoms of asthma and hay fever; while as an antipollutant it helps to eliminate toxic substances from the body.

Vitamin C is also responsible for tissue repair, the formation of antibodies and the stimulation of the white blood cells, as well as for the formation of the corticosteroid hormones in the adrenal glands.

It is probably the most researched antioxidant substance. Vitamin C is soluble in water and provides antioxidant protection for the watery compartments of our cells, tissues and organs. Our bodies cannot make ascorbate so we are dependent upon food sources for this vital nutrient. It is worth knowing that bioflavonoids usually occur alongside ascorbate and that they also have antioxidant properties.

Dr. Mark Levine, of the National Institute of Health (NIH) in the United States, has studied the effects of vitamin C on white blood cells. His work has shown that vitamin C is critical to the disease-fighting ability of white blood cells.

Research by Dr. Linus Pauling supports this conclusion. He found that the level of vitamin C in white blood cells is closely related to the body's ability to combat infection.

Vitamin C is found in citrus fruits, green vegetables, potatoes and fruit juice, so an adequate consumption of these foods will go a long way towards boosting the immune system.

ascorbate: Vitamin C

Vitamin E

Alpha tocopherol, to give vitamin E its other name, is a powerful nutrient which, in common with many other nutrients, is crucial for good health. As an enzyme-independent antioxidant, alpha tocopherol plays a particular role in protecting the fats in cell walls. (These fats, known as lipids, are particularly susceptible to oxidation by free radicals.)

As an antioxidant, alpha tocopherol has a myriad of vital functions. It stabilizes membranes and protects them against free radical damage. It protects the eyes, skin, liver, breast and calf muscle tissues and prevents tumor growth (associated with cancer).

Of particular importance is its ability to protect the lungs from oxidative damage (caused by air pollutants). It also protects and enhances the body's store of vitamin A. Vitamin E itself is enhanced by other antioxidants such as vitamin C and bioflavonoids such as Pycnogenol.

Foods rich in vitamin E include oils (wheatgerm, safflower, sunflower, soybean), nuts and seeds, asparagus, spinach, broccoli, butter, bananas, and strawberries.

Zinc

Zinc is found in alpha macroglobulin which is an important protein in the body's immune system. It follows that a shortage of the mineral will have severe consequences. What's more, zinc can actually help the immune system by clearing certain toxic metals from the body (cadmium and lead—present in car exhaust fumes).

Its presence is also essential for normal cell division and function and it has other cell-protecting properties apart from its antioxidant ones. In fact, zinc is involved in more enzymatic reactions than any other trace mineral.

Zinc is found in dairy products, beef, chicken, white fish and bread. It is an all-round valuable nutrient—so make sure your intake is satisfactory. A common sign of zinc deficiency is white marks on the fingernails.

Selenium

Its name derived from the moon goddess, Selene. This antioxidant trace mineral was first regarded as a poison until the discovery that it was actually needed to prevent liver tissue from degeneration.

Selenium is part of the enzyme glutathione peroxidase, which acts as an antioxidant. High doses of selenium, however, are toxic. Levels above 5 parts per million can be toxic.

Selenium and glutathione peroxidase levels are lower in patients with chronic pancreatitis and multiple sclerosis. Low selenium and glutathione peroxidase levels have been found in patients with Batten's disease, which is an inherited neurodegenerative disorder characterized by progressive loss of vision, epilepsy and dementia. Patients with asthma, Down's syndrome, and psoriasis have low blood selenium, which may aggravate their clinical characteristics. (Shamberger, R. J., "Selenium and the Antioxidant Defense System." *Journal of Advancement in Medicine.* [Spring 1992];5[1]:7–19.)

Evening Primrose Oil

The secret behind the oil of this unassuming flower lies in its gamma linolenic acid (GLA) content. Most vegetable oils contain linoleic acid which the body has to convert into GLA. People who are atopic (with allergic hypersensitivity) may be unable to convert linoleic acid into GLA. They are thought to be deficient in a particular enzyme that is needed for the conversion process. GLA in turn is used to produce a hormone-like anti-inflammatory substance called PGE1 (prostaglandin), which stimulates the T-suppressor cells that prevent the exaggerated immune response in atopic asthma and hay fever. The high content of GLA already present in evening primrose oil can shortcut the conversion process of linolenic acid into GLA and provide the GLA directly to the body, thereby boosting the formation of the PGE1.

From Pancreas:
→ large lobulated gland of vertebrates that secretes digestive enzymes and the hormones insuline and glucagon

? Pancreatitis

inflammation of the pancreas

Batten's disease = which is a inherited neuro degenerative disorder characterized by the progressive loss of vision, epilepsy and dementia.

Down's Syndrome!

Psoriasis

Multiple sclerosis: Demyelinating disease marked by hardened patches of brain tissues or the spinal cord and associated esp. with partial or complete paralysis and jerking muscle tremors

atopic: allergic hypersensitivity

GLA = Gamma Linolenic Acid
PGE1 = Prostaglanding

31

Chapter 7

Who Needs Pycnogenol?

TODAY, since many people forego fruits and vegetables, they stand to benefit from a concentrated nutritional supplement, like Pycnogenol.

Most of us will never be marooned on the ocean for months with contagious diseases constituting our major enemy. Nevertheless, we do face unheralded health risks, since we live longer and succumb principally to degenerative diseases, mostly self-inflicted, e.g. obesity, diabetes and osteoporosis.

There are particular groups of people who are in greater need of vitamin C than the rest of us. They include the elderly; those who are ill; pregnant or lactating women; athletes; smokers; people who drink a lot; those regularly on antibiotics, aspirin, the Pill and steroids; and diabetics.

People suffering any condition for which vitamin C and bioflavonoids have been recommended in the past might wish to give Pycnogenol a try as well—not instead of Vitamin C, however, since these products tend to reinforce one another, such that "the whole, exceeds the sum of the individual parts."

Pathogenesis = the origination and development of diseases [handwritten annotation]

The Elderly

In 1954, the free radical theory of aging was first described. It stated that a "single common process, modifiable by genetic and environmental factors, was responsible for ageing and death of all living things." Aging results from free radical reactions, which may be caused by the environment, from disease, and from intrinsic reaction within the aging process. There is an increasing number of studies which show that free radical reactions are involved in the pathogenesis of specific diseases. (Harman, Denham. "Free Radical Theory of Aging: History." In, Emerit, I., and Chance, B., *Free Radicals and Ageing*. Basel, Switzerland: Birkhauser Verlag, 1992; 1–10.)

Ample evidence shows that some antioxidants can delay the onset of many of the physical signs we have become conditioned to believe were intrinsic to the aging process. One theory that has been propounded for this is the fact that antioxidants have the ability to neutralize free radicals. You will remember that free radicals are a by-product of the breakdown of oxygen and that they have the potential to damage cells and tissues and DNA. The damage is repaired by the usual body processes, but over the years the damage builds up. Antioxidants can help to slow down the damage.

The elderly, particularly men living alone, are also at greater risk of developing scurvy because of the inadequacy of their diets. Scurvy is the disease of vitamin C deficiency. So, it obviously makes sense to supplement with vitamin C and its potentiator Pycnogenol for maximum benefit.

Vitamin C has been found to work well in conjunction with other antioxidant nutrients such as Vitamins A and E.

One study, reported in 1991, looked at thirty elderly institutionalized people. One group of them was given a placebo and the other group received a mixture of vitamins

Vitamin C with Vitamin A + E [handwritten annotation]

ACE

A, C and E. In terms of their nutritional status there was little real difference between the two groups. Neither group was deficient in vitamin E either before or after supplementation. Vitamin A levels improved slightly, and whereas before supplementation 22% were deficient in A, none were deficient afterwards. Interestingly, although vitamin C deficiency was the most common, deficiency levels of the vitamin didn't change much even after supplementation. What was noted, however, was that the workings of the immune system was enhanced. The number of T-cells increased significantly and the responsiveness of lymphocytes was stimulated, making these patients more resistant to illnesses. The authors of the report concluded that further studies would be beneficial to see if long-term supplementation made a difference to the death rates of such long-term institutionalized patients ("The Effect of Dietary Supplementation with Vitamins A, C and E on Cell-mediated Immune Function in Elderly Long-Stay Patients: A Randomized, Controlled Trial." In, Penn, N.D., et al, *Age and Ageing*, 1991; 20:169–174).

Another benefit of antioxidants for the elderly is their effect on blood cholesterol levels and the proportions of HDL (the "good" cholesterol) and LDL (the "bad"). As we age the proportion of HDL decreases. Vitamin C can help to increase the HDL cholesterol and so help to reduce the incidence of heart disease.

Since it is also the elderly who suffer most from hardening of the arteries and other circulatory problems due to vitamin C deficiency, there can be no doubt that supplementation would help to relieve much of the suffering endured by this section of our population.

In all the above, the importance of Pycnogenol lies in the fact that it is synergistic with vitamin C and is able to potentiate its antioxidant activity.

Synergistic: the interaction of discret agencies
(as industrial firms) agents (as drugs
From Synergism. or conditions such as
"the total effect is greater than the sum
of of the individual effect" ?
as 4 is greater than 1+2+3+4 ???
(as the effectiveness of a muscle with Pycnogenol)

34

When Ill

[handwritten annotations: ① vaccinia = cowpox ② the virus that produce or is the causative of the or causative agent of cowpox]

If you are ill the body uses up its reserves of vitamin C and so the need for the vitamin increases. The vitamin has also been found to inactivate viruses such as the herpes virus, hepatitis, polio, encephalitis, measles, pneumonia, and vaccinia. It does this by transforming oxygen molecules into molecules which attack the nucleic acid of the virus. It does the same thing to bacteria, including, for example, tuberculosis, tetanus, staphylococcus and typhoid.

Apart from going on the offensive, vitamin C also stimulates the production of interferon as well as white blood cells (leukocytes) which attack an invading organism.

A historic example of the benefits of vitamin C during illness was demonstrated by one study which compared the effects of treating ninety children with vitamin C against a control group of children receiving whooping cough vaccine. The vitamin C children had the vitamin administered orally or were injected. They were given 5,000 mg/day for seven days. The dosage was subsequently reduced until a level of 100 mg/day was reached. It was found that the illness lasted for only 1.5 to 2 days in the vitamin C children, whereas the average length of the illness in the vaccine children was 3 days. (*Journal of the American Medical Association.* [November 4, 1950]; as reported in *The Encyclopedia for Healthful Living.* Emmaus, PA: Rodale Books, 1994, p. 956.)

If you are hospitalized, having undergone surgery, your body's need for vitamin C will increase drastically. Not only will the body be fighting off possible infection, but the resistance to infection will be lowered. Vitamin C will stimulate the immune system and form part of the attack on any bacteria and viruses. It will speed wound healing by renewing the protein collagen needed for the repair of bones and the production of scar tissue.

RDA = Recommended

Some researchers suggest that surgery patients should consume about ten times the RDA (or 600 mg, slightly over the standard 500 mg supplement). Others believe that far higher amounts are needed. Such large doses are only possible through intravenous means, by-passing the body's digestive processes (although critically ill patients seem to have a tolerance to whatever amount of ascorbic acid their ailing bodies require). These amounts are in the tens of grams, rather than micrograms. Thirty grams would not be extraordinary according to these protocols, which is still about one ounce of ascorbic acid (5,000 times the RDA!).

The RDA, however, is often misinterpreted as a nutritional standard. Actually, it represents the minimum amount required from daily food by the majority of the population in order to remain disease free. It is not an optimal figure, nor a standard of safety or toxicity. Most healthy people can tolerate 5–10 grams without experiencing any gastro-intestinal upsets. Gradually building up the dose from that is achieved by afficionados of Pauling's regimen.

Vitamin C, especially with Pycnogenol, will, as part of its collagen-building function, strengthen capillary walls, which may help to prevent or reduce the incidence of varicose veins and stretch marks (by maintaining the elasticity of the skin).

Athletes

Correcting vitamin deficiencies in athletes can enhance performance, but those who are already nutrient sufficient have not shown improvement with vitamin megadoses. The use of antioxidant vitamins C and E, beta-carotene, zinc and selenium for athletes makes theoretical sense. Present studies from Australia and Great Britain evaluating the use of antioxidants in limiting muscle soreness and over-training will provide important data soon. Vitamin E dosage at 300 mgs per range, plus 2 gms of vitamin C and small doses of antioxidant minerals are really of no harm. The hope is that adequate antioxidant status will prevent muscle damage.

(Jancin, Bruce. "Sports Nutrition: What Works and What Doesn't." *Family Practice News*, September 15, 1993; 5.)

Adrenaline is manufactured by the body (in the adrenal glands) to prepare it for "fight or flight" in an emergency. It also helps the athlete to perform by raising blood pressure, quickening the heart rate and releasing glucose into the bloodstream, on the one hand, while on the other, slowing digestion. However, as adrenaline circulates in large amounts in the body, this can place a stress on the body— it is kept in a continual state of "fight or flight." The constant production of adrenaline can deplete the body's stores of vitamin C, and so it is advisable to replenish those stores by taking increased levels of vitamin C.

This scenario may also "ring" true for the busy executive, chained to his or her phone, putting out corporate "fires" all day long...except that the movement of the athlete releases the pent-up energies, whereas the sedentary executive must gradually process these substances over a much longer period of time. Indeed, with a daily job of extended hours and weekends, a busy executive will never catch up. That is why it is important to control stress. A little stimulation is an aid to performance, too much stimulation produces "burn-out" at best and well-known undesirable side-effects at worst (heart attacks, strokes etc.).

Common sports injuries are those annoying strains and sprains affecting muscles and joints, respectively. The resultant pain and swelling are debilitating. The mechanism of this is the same as that discussed for allergies, i.e. a histamine reaction. Hence, Pycnogenol reduces inflammation for athletes, even if they don't suffer from asthma!

Professor Masquelier undertook a study with soccer players in 1983. Immediately after the injury, the players were placed on a descending protocol of Pycnogenol supplementation, beginning at 400 mg and ending after 10 days with 200 mg. The Pycnogenol group showed greatly reduced inflammation compared with the placebo (sugar pill) group.

We can review Dr. Bucci's thoroughly researched recommendations, as well as touch upon long-term, chronic problems, such as arthritis and pain (especially from team contact sports like football) which tend to play a big part in the later years of many athletes. *(Bucci, Luke. Nutrition Applied to Injury Rehabilitation and Sports Medicine. Boca Raton, FL: C.R.C. Press, 1992.)*

For acute joint trauma (including sprains and strains) Dr. Bucci recommends an initial phase of treatment consisting of:

> Proteolytic enzymes
> Vitamin C
> Bioflavonoids and
> Curcumin (Turmeric).

Vitamin C and citrus bioflavonoids are the best known antioxidants, although Dr. Bucci also provides an extended list for an even more potent antioxidant mixture: Beta-carotene, vitamin E, selenium and cysteine.

Bruises require a similar treatment protocol:

> Proteolytic enzymes
> Vitamin C
> Bioflavonoids and
> Antioxidant mixture.

Fractures have the same basic requirement, with the addition of:

> Glucosamines and
> Chondroitin sulfates.

Lacerations and wounds, once more, have the same basic requirement, together with vitamin A and zinc.

> Proteolytic enzymes
> Vitamin C
> Bioflavonoids

Antioxidant mixture
Curcumin (Turmeric)
Vitamin A and
Zinc.

Vitamin C

Due in large part to the work of the late Dr. Linus Pauling, vitamin C is the most widely consumed vitamin supplement among athletes.

Famous as the antidote for scurvy, vitamin C is noted in college textbooks for its role in collagen synthesis. Current interest surrounds its use as an antioxidant. It takes only 30 mg of vitamin C to prevent scurvy, so this is the level set by a number of RDA boards around the world. The US has been more generous (60 mg), but even elder-medical statesmen like Dr. Kenneth Cooper of the Aerobics Center, the founder of the aerobics movement, have come around to the conclusion that everyone, especially athletes, requires more antioxidants. Pauling used to recommend building up tolerance in order to achieve a maintenance intake around 20 gms daily which served him into his nineties. The Colgan Institute uses 2–12 gms. Many athletes self-administer higher doses at the first sign of a cold. So-called toxic levels (actually usually no more than an intolerance), produce some gastrointestinal disturbances. Serious injuries and diseases may require the administration of larger doses intravenously, although this remains controversial.

Critics, none of whom can boast double individual Nobel prizes, warn of interference with copper and iron status, kidney stones, gout and complicated pregnancy. The Pauling Institute continues to research vitamin C and has accumulated a mammoth body of research.

Smokers

It is well known that smokers expose themselves (and others) to the risk of developing cancers and heart and arterial disease. They may also suffer from smoker's cough (a sign that the body is trying to rid itself of the toxins released by cigarette smoke), chronic bronchitis, emphysema, indigestion, peptic ulcers, conjunctivitis as well as partial sight loss. For smokers there is also a greater risk of infertility, impotence and miscarriage. Babies and young children can also be affected by their parents' smoking.

Cigarette smoke contains a number of toxins—the main culprits being nicotine, carbon monoxide and tar as well as toxic heavy metals and low level radioactive isotopes. Research has shown that smokers' levels of nutrients are severely depleted, particularly the antioxidant nutrients—vitamins C and E and beta carotene. In the battle against excessive free radicals these nutrients are burned up. In fact, "vitamin C hypovitaminosis is the most frequent nutritional deficiency among smokers," according to an article in *Family Practice News*, August 1–14, 1990;20 (15): 29.

Not only is there a decrease in antioxidant nutrients, but smoking increases plasma levels in the blood and creates favorable conditions for the oxidation of the "bad" cholesterol LDL which, in turn, affect the arterial walls causing them to harden. There is also a greater incidence of lesions.

Since the respiratory burst reaction may cause an oxidative stress in smokers, in one study they were supplemented for ten days with the antioxidants L-selenium-methionine, vitamins E and C, and beta-carotene. After ten days of supplementation with these antioxidants, respiratory burst reaction of smokers was significantly decreased by 20 to 75%. The study concluded that, since oxidative stress associated with the respiratory burst reaction may cause autodigestive reactions in the lungs of smokers, it may be recommended that smokers use high doses of antioxidants to inhibit these pathological changes. (Clausen, Jorgen. "The Influence of Antioxidants on the Enhanced Respiratory Burst Reaction in Smokers." *Beyond Deficiency: New Views on the Function and Health Effects of Vitamins*. New York: Academy of Sciences, February 9-12, 1992, p. 7.)

In addition, nicotine causes the overproduction of adrenaline and speeds up the heart rate so that there is an increase in blood pressure. Studies are confirming that vitamin C supplementation lowers the heart rate and blood pressure and that this effect is greater when more vitamin C is consumed. Suffice it to say, there is more than one reason why Pycnogenol supplementation would be advisable for smokers and for those who use tobacco in other forms.

Alcohol

If you drink heavily then you are putting yourself at risk of developing not just cirrhosis of the liver, which is the most well known of the alcohol-related diseases, but also cancer of the esophagus and mouth, heart failure, damaged kidneys, mental illness, brain damage, strokes, high blood pressure, impotence in men, and low birthweight babies in women.

The B-group of vitamins are particularly important in counteracting the consequences of alcohol abuse, but vitamin C supplementation is also important. Alcohol drinkers are likely to be deficient, as alcohol interferes with the body's absorption of vitamin C. What vitamin C is absorbed is used up in the fight against the toxic effects of the alcohol.

Professor Vincent Zannoni of the University of Michigan Medical School revealed, in 1986, that the vitamin may help to prevent the fat build-up in the liver which can precipitate cirrhosis. This was demonstrated both in guinea pigs and in humans. He recommended a vitamin C intake of 5g/day for people who drink up to the equivalent of three beers a day.

People who smoke and drink are only compounding their health problems. It seems that the interaction of the components in cigarette smoke and in alcohol give rise to the development of acetaldehyde which plays a part in lung diseases, alcoholic degeneration of the brain, and alcoholic heart disease. Dr. Herbert Sprince of Jefferson Medical College administered large amounts of vitamin C together with thiamine (a B vitamin) and found that it gave some protection against the effects of acetaldehyde.

Therefore, it is all the more important that Pycnogenol be included in the supplement regimen.

Medication

If you have been taking antibiotics over a period of time, or cortisone, aspirin and other painkilling drugs, your levels of vitamin C may have been depleted since these drugs can interfere with the absorption of the vitamin. Some drugs can even cause the body to excrete vitamin C two or three times more than normal. Apart from that, prolonged use of antibiotics can actually have a deleterious effect on the immune system in that not only do they kill off harmful bacteria but they may start killing off friendly bacteria which form a part of the body's arsenal against illness. If the immune system is weakened then we become susceptible to infection. Optimal amounts of vitamin C are vital to ensure the efficient functioning of the immune system. To potentiate this it is well worth considering Pycnogenol supplementation together with vitamin C. Indeed, although Dr. Pauling always recommended a cheap form of ascorbic acid powder as the key source, vulnerable people may wish to obtain vitamin C which also contains some bioflavonoids, as well as consume fruits and raw fruit juices.

More than one researcher has bemoaned the recent loss of Dr. Linus Pauling who pioneered research into vitamin C. Famous for encouraging hundreds of thousands of people around the globe to take vitamin C to stave off a cold, the

Pauling Institute went on to conduct extensive research into other uses for vitamin C, including cancer and AIDS.

Pauling enjoyed a vigorous lifestyle into his nineties, finally succumbing to prostate cancer. Would prostate cancer have been fatal much earlier had he not supplemented (about 18 grams daily) for most of his life? Would his life have remained cancer-free with more diverse supplementation?

We may never know the answers to these questions, for Dr. Pauling, or on an individual basis for anyone. However, as more people consume Pycnogenol we may be able to identify trends in epidemiological terms (i.e., over populations of hundreds of thousands of people) by shifts of a point or two.

These shifts may be most obvious for the leading killer diseases like heart disease. However, smaller groups, even breast cancer or prostate cancer, may be more difficult to monitor, especially over the short term. Changes in lifestyle and nutrition may need to be implemented at an early age to completely offset any developmental links to disease.

It is not beyond the realms of possibility that the impact of fetal nutrition (via the pregnant mother) is critical, together with consistent adherence to the same level of nutrient intake over a lifetime (the next hundred years?). Thus it would take a century for any meaningful results to "come in."

Those of us who do not want to wait a hundred years should consider that we are each an experiment of one anyway! It seems reasonable, since there is no known contra-indication, or toxicity involved, provided that the disposable income is available, to give Pycnogenol a trial for a few months and see if any benefit is perceptible.

Of course, testing the limits for any "miracle" nutrient is not recommended. Washing a few vitamins down as an antidote with your morning coffee, after habitually smoking packages of cigarettes and sinking into alcoholic oblivion, is likely to be doomed to failure! Even switching to red wine will not provide the benefits of its constituents in direct proportion to consumption; there will be "diminishing marginal returns."

On the other hand, including Pycnogenol as a supplement to a balanced diet after giving up smoking and drinking is likely to prove to be beneficial. The so-called French paradox is the best known example. The French enjoy low rates of heart disease in comparison to other Western nations, in spite of high fat consumption and gourmet meals. The "secret" seems to be the antioxidant properties contained within the red wine, i.e. the same factors as Pycnogenol, rather than the alcohol itself.

Summary

Individuals who may wish to take a hard look at the potential benefits of supplementing with Pycnogenol include:

- middle-aged, older segments of the population;
- those who do not eat sufficient fruits and vegetables;
- those with "Western" diseases: obesity, diabetes and osteoporosis;
- patients with other degenerative diseases e.g. arthritis;
- families with a high incidence of cancer;
- drug addicts (both prescription, e.g. antibiotics, anti-inflammatories) and recreational (including alcohol and cigarettes);
- individuals in extreme lifestyles, less likely to be explorers crossing the ocean but those who train for fitness in an intense manner, on a daily basis, throughout the year;
- anyone with a compromised immune system, vulnerable to infections e.g. asthmatics, yeast infections ("candida");

- combinations of the above, e.g. female members of families with a history of breast cancer; men whose relatives have had prostate problems with advancing age (i.e. almost everyone!).

Chapter 8

Other Therapeutic Uses

A recent book, by chiropractic physician, James D. Krystosik, states that Pycnogenol is effective against sixty diseases; the book then lists about half of them. The major author in this field, Richard A. Passwater, Ph.D. refers to eighty diseases (seventy of them free radical related) and lists about a quarter of them. A comprehensive listing is included in this chapter.

The inference is clear, there are certain main benefits of Pycnogenol which translate to particular disease categories; and if one wanted to, one could expand upon each heading with numerous sub-divisions.

Thus, while Pycnogenol is well known for its beneficial effect on the heart, one must not ignore the attendant vascular system, which includes a second major organ—the lungs—but also encompasses the skeleton and spleen where some blood cells originate. Furthermore, oxygenated blood reaches, quite literally, every cell in the body. Therefore, every system, indeed every class of cells, may also be itemized, in some way, as dependent upon an adequate supply of nutrients, specifically, Pycnogenol™. Every disease associated with any of these components could, then, be justifiably enumerated.

While the research has not yet been conclusive with regard to most of the conditions listed, several key areas have been extensively researched. These will be featured herein.

Vitamin C has been investigated over a longer period of time, and intensively, largely due to the efforts of Dr. Linus Pauling. Vitamin C has been shown to help in virtually all of the following conditions. As a Vitamin C potentiator, Pycnogenol supplementation can reasonably be expected to make a positive contribution for this reason alone.

AIDS

Reports at the ninth International Conference on AIDS in Berlin, Germany, found early AZT confers no clear survival benefit. Antioxidants such as N-acetylcysteine can prevent apoptosis, which programs cell death. Oxidative stress can mediate apoptosis. In HIV infection, apoptosis is a permanent and chronic situation. Dr. Montagnier is planning trials with other antioxidants to see if they help prevent apoptosis when combined with antiretroviral drugs. He stated it would not be a bad idea for HIV infected patients to take antioxidants. (McKeown, L.A. "HIV Pioneer Eyes Antioxidants." *Medical Tribune.* [June 24, 1993];34 [12]:1, 8.)

In HIV infection, the altered immune system has difficulty reacting to the increased free radical oxygen release. There is an overall antioxidant deficiency in HIV infection due to impaired scavenging systems, altered structure and function of the alimentary tract which can result in achlorhydria, malabsorption, loss of mucosal integrity and loss of appetite secondary to chronic nutritional deficiencies. In preliminary work, the antioxidants vitamin A and C have shown efficacy in HIV infection. Phytopharmaceuticals are an important source of antioxidant compounds. Plant elements with antioxidant activity include enzymes like catalases, peroxidases and superoxide dismutase. Carotenoids are some of the most studied plant-derived products having antioxidant capability. Vitamin C, glycosides and phospholipids have additional antioxidant protection.

(Greenspan, H.C. "The Role of Reactive Oxygen Species, Antioxidants and Phytopharmaceuticals in Human Immunodeficiency Virus Activity." *Medical Hypotheses*. [1993]; 40:85–92.)

Allergy

Allergies are thought by many to be a "plague" brought on by modern civilization, or, more specifically, the synthetic ingredients contained within the air we breathe, the water we drink and the foods we eat.

Lending credence to this viewpoint is the medical history that cannot identify any semblance of an allergic reaction until the industrial era, together with recent increases in the incidence of allergies, such that every family in America seems to be affected to some extent.

Common symptoms of allergies (sneezing, runny nose, watery eyes) are triggered by histamine. Reimann has shown in rat studies that Pycnogenol significantly reduces the formation of histamine, thereby reducing symptoms. Anecdotal reports from consumers of Pycnogenol products seem to support the animal studies, although, of course, the conclusive medical studies will not be undertaken in America so long as Pycnogenol does not have to fulfill the requirements reserved for drugs by the FDA. It is just too expensive and time-consuming. Anyway, the bottom-line is that each of us is an "experiment of one," and we must try it for ourselves and assess its efficacy in our own particular condition, rather than hoping to be one of the 60% of people who have been shown to benefit in a "double-blind" placebo-controlled scientific study of hundreds of thousands of other people, none of whom, or even some of whom, may have a remotely similar physiological profile to your own.

Histamine is a potent inflammatory chemical released by specialized "mast" cells in response to the presence of a foreign body in the blood. Keahey has suggested that Pycnogenol works by preventing the breakdown of the mast cells. It would seem that suppressing a natural reaction might make the body more vulnerable to the foreign intruder. Alternatively, the mast cells may be spared through other mechanisms, such as the interception of some of these substances by other systems, presumably reinforced by Pycnogenol. Or it may be that Pycnogenol defuses the situation by weakening these agents in some way, possibly through its antioxidant properties, working at the electron level (i.e. free radicals).

Pycnogenol has become a standard form of treatment for hay fever in Finland. However, allergies are now linked to other conditions, far beyond grass pollen, extending to hyperactivity (attention-deficit disorder) in children. Moreover, other problems may develop in adults which give no clue to their underlying basis as an allergic reaction to some chemical: anxiety, colitis, compulsive drinking, depression, fatigue, headaches and high blood pressure. A whole new sub-specialty in medicine, environmental health, or clinical ecology, has developed in response to the growing demand for allergy specialists, as well as the growing number of patients who seem to find little or no relief from standard treatment protocols for their presenting symptoms. No headache pill will end frequent headaches if the source of the problem is a commonplace chemical, e.g. chlorine in tap water, or corn syrup in foods. These medical specialists have an index of suspicion to go along with their range of sensitivity tests so that they may permanently cure the cause, rather than only temporarily alleviate the symptom.

Many patients are grateful that someone finally believes them and offers a solution rather than writing them off as having a psychiatric problem ("malingerer," "hypochondriac," etc.). The classic example is probably the unfortunate female patient who experiences all sorts of gynecological problems. Even the surgical solution is named after the perception that a complaining female is *hysterical*, i.e., *hyster-ectomy* is the solution to all female ills. In fact, the solution for some may be as simple as avoiding certain chemicals in feminine hygiene products.

Arthritis

Arthritis is an umbrella term for over two hundred different forms of the disease which affects collagen, the protein glue which holds us all together. The two most widely known and most commonly treated forms are rheumatoid arthritis and osteoarthritis. All of the forms exhibit joint inflammation as a symptom. This results in pain, swelling, and stiffness of the joints. Sometimes the joints become fused and deformed.

Osteoarthritis is the result of the cartilage surrounding the joints wearing away over the years. Degeneration of the cartilage is thought to be due to a biochemical abnormality in the metabolism of the tissue. The damaged cartilage leaves the bone exposed and this develops rough projections which in turn cause friction between the bones. It is this that gives rise to the inflammation and consequent pain and stiffness. The symptoms are usually to be found in the knee, hips and spine, as well as, occasionally, the hand.

Rheumatoid arthritis, although its symptoms may be similar, has actually been described as an autoimmune disease in which the immune system turns attacker and manufactures antibodies against its own tissues.

The two other most common forms of arthritis are ankylosing spondylitis which originates in the immune system but affects the spinal vertebrae, and gout.

The conventional treatment for arthritis is the prescription of nonsteroidal anti-inflammatory drugs (NSAIDs). They deal with the symptoms, however, but not the fundamental cause.

Vitamin C is beneficial for all types of arthritis. In its capacity as an antistress nutrient it can help to combat the stress which causes tense muscles and increases pain. Where blood levels of the vitamin are high the lubrication fluid between the joints (synovial fluid) becomes thinner and this also helps to relieve pain. Studies in which patients were administered 6g/day of vitamin C brought about "astonishing results." Its properties for revitalizing the immune system are relevant here, too. Further, it has been found that high levels of vitamin C can help to ward off the crippling effects of the disease. This is because of the vitamin's vital role in the formation of collagen which is essential for healthy joints.

When used in cases of arthritis, Taxifolin, a component found in Pycnogenol, was found to possess significant anti-inflammatory activities similar to hydrocortisone. Proanthocyanidin was about twice as effective as phenylbutazone (used to treat arthritis, bursitis, etc.) without the toxic side effects. It is not known whether proanthocyanidins act as a palliative mechanism or actually reverse the underlying disease process. ("Anti-inflammatory and anti-allergic properties of flavonoids." In, Gabor, M., *Progress in Clinical and Biological Research, USA* vol. 213, pp. 471–480.)

Burns

Vitamin C is required for the formation of collagen—main protein component of fibrous and scar tissue needed to heal burns. Further, the stress of injury creates a higher demand for vitamin C. Pycnogenol can help by potentiating the effects of vitamin C.

Cancer Prevention

Antioxidants are believed to offer protection against the risk of most cancers. A study on "Antioxidant Intake in the United States," (reported in *Toxicology and Industrial Health* [1993]; 9[1/2], 295–301) evaluated antioxidant intake (vitamin C, E and carotenoids) from foods and vitamin supplements. This study reports that many Americans are consuming levels of antioxidant nutrients considerably below the optimal level to prevent chronic diseases. The problem is especially significant for those near the poverty level. Even for those 300% above the poverty level, 75% consume less than the RDA for vitamin E, 25% consumed less than the RDA for vitamin C. This underlines the case for supplementation for antioxidant nutrients like Pycnogenol.

Capillary Resistance

Capillary resistance is an aspect of blood circulation; one could say "microcirculation," which is why it is so often overlooked. The doctor must become suspicious about it while the patient will usually be oblivious to it. Basically, it concerns the ability of the blood supply to pass through the entire network of blood vessels providing oxygen and other nutrients to every cell in the body. Any interference with this process causes impaired function at the cellular level. This may be associated with peripheral areas like the hands, feet and ears, which may change appearance but usually this will only be noticeable by others, e.g. "Your hands are cold!" or "When did you develop a crease in your earlobe?"

As the famed aerobics expert, Dr. Kenneth Cooper, is fond of reminding us, "The first sign of heart disease is often death." The American Heart Association cautions us that high blood pressure is a "silent" but "deadly" disease, to encourage us to have our blood pressure taken. Otherwise we go about our daily lives oblivious to the problem; we are "an accident waiting for a place to happen."

Specifically, at the capillary level the exchange of nutrients and waste products takes place. Capillary resistance measures the force required before fluids and red blood cells will leak out through a capillary. Machines are available, operating essentially in the same manner as a "Love Bite" such that a vacuum is applied until bruising marks appear at the surface. The stronger the suction required the higher the resistance, or the more intact the collagen fibers forming the capillary walls are. Dr. Richard A. Passwater has delineated three contributions made by Pycnogenol to this process: Pycnogenol contributes initially in support of vitamin C to the formation of collagen which makes up both the single cell walls of the capillaries and the intercellular matrix; it reinforces the collagen fibers directly; and it provides protection against free radical attack.

Other circulatory problems develop and manifest themselves in more obvious ways. Diabetics realize there is a visual problem when they lose vision through leakage of the blood vessels within the eye (diabetic retinopathy); other people are horrified to find lumpy (varicose) veins along their legs, especially if they are young females, seeking to follow revealing fashion trends of short skirts and sheer hose. Each of these problems deserves to be treated separately.

Suffice to say, for the moment, that Pycnogenol has been indicated to benefit all of the circulatory processes involved in preventing these problems, or reducing these problems once they have developed. With Pycnogenol usage, blood moves more freely throughout the body.

Cataract Prevention

As an antioxidant, vitamin C can offer protection against the risk of cataract formation One study evaluated forty-seven patients for over fifteen years for the relationship between antioxidant vitamin status and senile cataracts. Low serum concentrations of the antioxidant vitamins predicted the development of senile cataract patients. (Knekt, P., et al, "Serum Antioxidant Vitamins and Risk of Cataract." BMJ, [1992]; 305:1392–1394.)

Cholesterol

It may be news to many people that cholesterol is not just an indicator of the excess consumption of fatty foods! The body, in fact, produces more cholesterol than most of us could consume if we binged on fried chicken and donuts all day long. Recent research has revealed the mystery why the body should produce an excess of a product which then blocks the arteries and can result in "homo-suicide."

Two major mechanisms appear to be at work. First, while we have concentrated upon different forms of cholesterol—high density, low density, very low density (good and bad, respectively)—the main factor may be whether the cholesterol is in good condition or has been ravaged by the free radicals at large within the body, i.e. "oxidized" and forming "foam cells."

What maintains the natural state of cholesterol so that it performs its normal functions? You guessed it—Pycnogenol (and, of course, other antioxidants).

Since we have just discussed blood circulation, the second mechanism may be more readily understood: we have always bemoaned the formation of "hardened arteries."

The cholesterol plaque laid down restricts the circulation of blood and oxygen; in particular, if the plaque breaks off and is carried to the brain, it causes a stroke; and if the circulation to the heart is eliminated, it causes a heart attack ("myocardial infarction," i.e. death of the heart muscle denied oxygen by the loss of its normal supply system).

Recent research by Dr. Matthias Rath has provided a new perspective to this problem. It is not that there is just too much cholesterol, so that the body doesn't have a means of coping with it and thus stores it along the blood vessel walls as the elimination highways are backed up. No. This storing effect is a normal process which is designed to reinforce faulty walls, leaking blood. Therefore, it is not sufficient to merely reduce cholesterol intake, one must provide the missing nutrients which provide the nutrients required by the blood vessel walls to maintain normal function.

You're jumping ahead....Yes, one important factor in maintaining the integrity of the blood vessel walls is Pycnogenol.

Dr. David White of England's Nottingham University has pioneered this field, reporting his findings at medical conferences only as recently as 1990. He has referred to Pycnogenol as the "atherosclerosis antidote"! (Atherosclerosis is the plaque formation in blood vessels, like the build-up in water pipes in hard water areas, the so-called "hardened artery.")

For some time epidemiologists have observed that wine consumers have received some kind of special protection against heart disease, the so-called "French paradox" (gourmet foods, wine and low levels of cardiovascular disease). Dr. White has found that it is not the alcohol per se which is imparting these benefits but the special factors in red wine, the bioflavonoids (like Pycnogenol™). White wine doesn't contain these same special factors.

Cardiologists have routinely prescribed aspirin to reduce blood clotting but the gastrointestinal side-effects from excessive use has brought this practice into question. They might well do better to switch their allegiance to Pycnogenol as it imparts the same basic benefits (together with some additional ones) without the undesirable side-effects.

Sadly, Pycnogenol is not a drug, even of the over-the-counter variety, so the mainstream of the medical establishment will probably eschew it in spite of its claims, no doubt on the grounds that it hasn't undergone the scientific trials, etc. The pro-active patient will have to make a lot of noise and do a lot of searching if medical assent is deemed necessary.

Other people may just try Pycnogenol on the basis of the scientific studies reported from Europe and the overwhelming, anecdotal reports from their peers. The same has been true for vitamin C.

Interestingly, physicians who have spent decades adhering to the establishment views are beginning to be convinced by the evidence on antioxidants. Dr. Kenneth Cooper is perhaps the best known example. Author of many books, Cooper has just published his latest on the subject of antioxidants, recommending vitamins A (in the form of beta-carotene), C and E.

Do not make the mistaken assumption that the story of Pycnogenol is intended to promote the use of Pycnogenol as the pre-eminent antioxidant, over and above all others. In fact, Pycnogenol enhances the action of vitamin C which, in its turn, regenerates vitamin E. It is not wise to search for the Magic Pill—all of the antioxidants work together. The whole range, from A through C to E together with the associated plant-derived bioflavonids (which include Pycnogenol™), works together synergistically to provide the best protection against free radicals.

Diabetic Retinopathy

One of the most common causes of blindness today is the micro-bleeding which affects the fragile capillaries in the eyes of adult diabetics. In France, following the pioneering work by Dr. G. Maynard, Pycnogenol is now the treatment of choice among many ophthalmologists.

Dr. Maynard prescribed a loading dose of 80–120 mg of Pycnogenol for the first week and a maintenance dose of 40–80 mg for the remainder of the month (up to four months). Fully 90% of the patients showed significant improvement in their visual acuity.

At the University of Wurzburg in Germany, Dr. Leydhecker achieved results with Pycnogenol comparable to the best drug available (Dexium, calcium dobesilate) for retarding the progression of diabetic retinopathy. The study covered a period of six months.

Edema

Vitamin C with bioflavonoids helps prevent the capillary weakness which allows fluid to leak out from the bloodstream into the body tissue thereby causing swelling of hands and feet.

Swollen legs are another form of circulatory impairment, i.e. the blood flow pools as the body lacks the ability to overcome gravity. A study at the University of Florence, Italy has illustrated the effects of Pycnogenol on edema. Forty subjects (thirteen men and twenty-seven women) between the ages of thirty and seventy were divided into two groups. One group received 300 mg of Pycnogenol for a period of sixty days while the other group, which served as a control group, was given a placebo supplement. After the first thirty days, scientists observed that 26% of those taking Pycnogenol had their swellings reduced. At sixty days, 63% of the participants were free from swelling in their legs. Eleven percent of those on the supplement reported a decrease in the feeling of heaviness in their legs after thirty days and this figure went up to 33% after sixty days.

Further, 38% of those taking Pycnogenol reported a total relief from pain after thirty days. This percentage rose to 67% after a period of sixty days. (Report from Prof. Arcangeli, University of Florence, June 1989.)

A case report from Dr. Krystosik cites the benefit of Pycnogenol in improving circulation and energy levels in an elderly lady within a period of three weeks. (Krystosik, James D., D.C. *Pycnogenol. Nature's Prescription for Aging, Allergies...* Garrettsville, OH: Good News Press, 1995.)

Premenstrual Syndrome

PMS affects about one-third of women and is attributed to fluctuating hormone levels.

Professor Masquelier reports a 1987 study in which 165 women were provided 200 mg of Pycnogenol per day during the second half of their monthly cycle. Symptoms were relieved in 67% of the women by the third month and 80% by the fourth cycle. Additionally, 67% also reported relief of dysmenorrhea (period pains). (Masquelier, J. et al, *OPC in Practice*, Alpha Omega Publishers, 1993.) Apparently, the hormone theory needs to be replaced with that of free radicals.

Prostate

Anecdotal reports are not usually valued very highly in medical circles. However, when doctors themselves benefit from nutrition supplements, they tend to become firm believers, and even credible sources. One such example is the case of Dr. W. Lamar Rosquist of Salt Lake City. He suffered with BPH (benign prostatic hypertrophy, i.e. a swollen prostate gland) which is very common in older men. It was embarrassing for him to leave patients in order to go to the bathroom so frequently.

Dr. Rosquist resorted to Pycnogenol for six months without enjoying any significant benefit. Then he read about calculating the dosage based upon body weight and increased his intake to 11 × 20 mg tablets daily (taken six in the morning and the remaining five in the evening). After one week he enjoyed an uninterrupted night of sleep. Bliss for such sufferers!

Skin Cancer

At the Second International Conference on Melanoma in October of 1989 it was accepted that the main cause of melanoma in Caucasians was exposure to sunlight, especially UVB. Good antioxidant status, especially with regards to vitamins A, C and E, and the trace element selenium are important in cellular antioxidant systems. (Mackie, Bruce S.,

Dr. and Leila E. Mackie. "Prevention of Melanoma." *Nutrition and Cancer* [1990]; 14[2]: 81–83.)

In the plant kingdom, plant phenols are also believed to provide a chemical defense against UV (ultra-violet) radiation.

Sick Child Syndrome

Several medical practitioners are suspecting that the "sick child syndrome"—whereby the child requires antibiotics as an infant, eventually has ear tubes to achieve drainage, develops asthma and loses other surplus organs (tonsils, adenoids, appendix) along the way—may, in fact, merely require support for a compromised immune system! Pycnogenol is being increasingly recommended. Additionally, "radical" pediatricians have been substituting Echinacea (an herbal remedy) for antibiotics, as their concerns have grown over the dwindling efficacy of antibiotics and the ever-growing resistance of the bacteria they used to easily control.

Thus, as children under the "high-tech" care of modern medicine have become sicker the possibility is being appreciated that the "high tech" solution may, in fact, be part of the problem. As children are exposed to antibiotics, their own immune system is compromised; while their potential to fight-off infection is decreased, the strength of that infection is increased. With each new infection, they slide further down the slippery slope of "high tech" medicine, facing a "lose-lose" predicament from which there seems to be no solution, other than to search for an alternative system of care! The more infections and treatments they undergo, the weaker and sicker they become. Pycnogenol can represent a first step in the right direction towards building up a child's natural immune defenses.

The growing list of conditions which, although previously unsuspected, are now shown to have their roots in allergy, indicates that allergic reactions comprise more than simple sneezes and wheezes. Allergies need not begin in childhood, nor can people rely upon "out-growing" them. Asthma is becoming an increasingly fatal disease, in spite of the proliferation of inhalers and inhalants to combat it. Nor does age necessarily guarantee immunity! Even though the skin and lungs are the first barriers (and usually the first to fall) against an allergen attack, virtually any part of the body is vulnerable. Once the defenses have been breached, muscles, joints, veins and even the brain, the command system of the body, can fall victim to invasion.

Just like the Roman Empire of old, or the Russian Empire of recent years, collapse does not occur because the outside foe is irresistible and forces its way in. The "foe is irresistible" only because the body is unable to resist in the normal manner. Chronic disease is predominantly a "collapse" from within. Pycnogenol serves to reinforce the body's own defenses.

Skin Eruptions

A consumer magazine (*Total Health*, February, 1995) related the story of Dorothy who had fought a skin eruption battle for nine years. Her legs, including her hips and thighs, were covered with itchy bumps and oozing sores. All sorts of tests, lotions and elimination diets were tried, to no avail.

At the instigation of a friend, Dorothy finally bought some Pycnogenol at the local health food store and, amazingly, improved within a week.

The skin we think of, generally, is just the outer layer of the body's largest organ. It is just a layer of dead cells! Underneath, the living tissue is made up of a fibrous protein ("collagen") which contains vitamin C, and its production is potentiated by Pycnogenol.

Pycnogenol circulates in the blood before arriving in the dermis where it remains for around seventy-two hours before being eliminated via perspiration and urination. While there, it has performed wonders for acne, allergic rashes, bed sores, burns, eczema and psoriasis.

Stress

Hardly a moment goes by when we are not subject to some form of stress. It may be emotional. You may be suffering from a major life trauma such as a relationship breakdown, a bereavement, financial worries or redundancy. Or your stress may come from the minutiae of life with which you are continually bombarded. There are physical stresses, too. Your office may be poorly ventilated; you may be subjected to electromagnetic waves from VDUs or overhead power cables, cigarette smoke or food additives. All of these factors, and more, can take their toll and produce the symptoms which we call stress.

These symptoms may take the form of behavioral problems, or feelings of depression and anxiety, to a lowering of our resistance to illness. Stress factors result in the release of the chemicals adrenaline and noradrenaline. The heart rate increases, blood pressure is raised, blood is diverted from the skin and digestive organs to the muscles, glucose is released and the body is ready to fight or to flee.

These mechanisms are essential to our survival in an emergency and are resolved by physical activity. Most of the stresses that we encounter, however, do not require us to act physically and so the mechanisms do not have the opportunity to wind down. We remain in a state of near constant state of "fight or flight." If we are continually assailed by stress factors which do not find an outlet, this can, over a period of time, affect many of our body processes.

We may end up suffering from elevated blood pressure, ulcers, diarrhea and gastric upsets. Tension in the muscles and joints may later give rise to arthritis, backache, muscular aches and pains. Those people who have a tendency to anxiety and depression may find these conditions exacerbated. The immune system is compromised and its ability to resist infection, tissue degeneration and cancerous cells is reduced. Enzyme systems which control the activities of our cells are impaired. The aging process is accelerated. Stress also depletes the body's stores of nutrients, thereby increasing the body's requirements.

Obviously, solutions should be sought to resolve the personal difficulties that cause stress; and the harmful eating and drinking habits, and smoking, that adversely affect our nutrient levels should be discontinued. Exercise and relaxation can also help to reduce internal tension. Antistress nutrients should also be used.

Vitamin C (together with bioflavonoids) is known as the "antistress" nutrient. It helps in a variety of ways. First, it can detoxify the body. One experiment conducted at the University of Queensland in Australia involved exposing mice to different concentrations of ozone (which, as you know, is a component of smog) over a period of thirty minutes. Fifty percent of the vitamin C in the lung tissue of the mice was found to be used up in combating the ozone. The researchers concluded that the vitamin C in the lung itself was the preventive factor. This shows the importance of making sure that the body tissues are saturated with the vitamin.

Secondly, vitamin C can help to maintain energy. It has been demonstrated that increasing vitamin C intake can cause a corresponding increase in how much glycogen is stored in the muscles and the liver. We need glycogen for storing energy. Other research has focused on whether vitamin C can reduce fatigue. Dr. Emanuel Cheraskin, professor and chairman of the Department of Oral Medicine at the University of Alabama, conducted a survey of over four hundred people. When comparing vitamin C intake with symptoms of fatigue it was found that the 330 people who consumed more than 400 mg/day had a "fatigue score" of half that of the rest who consumed less than 100 mg/day. The vitamin may help to keep people alert, too. In a study of coal miners, fewer accidental injuries being reported when certain of them received supplements of vitamin C.

Varicose Veins

Besides the well-known cosmetic features of varicose veins, sufferers usually also find they experience symptoms including aching, itching, burning and fatigue. Varicose veins also correlate closely (even if they can't be shown to directly cause) with other cardiovascular problems, like thrombophlebitis, pulmonary embolism, heart attacks and strokes.

Essentially, the return journey of the blood to the heart, which is against the flow of gravity, is aided by a system of locks, like canal systems. In this process, the blood is supported by semilunar valves in sections, so that the body does not have to pump against the full length of the body at once. However, if the valve in one section collapses, the vein will bulge as the next section pools into it; then the subjacent valve must support more than double the normal load. Hence, it will likely fail next. And so on.

Dr. G. Fume-Haake in Hamburg, Germany, conducted a study with one hundred ten people, forty-one of whom also reported night leg cramp problems. A daily dose of Pycnogenol (90 mg) was given. Significant improvement was evident in 77% of the group. Within the subgroup with leg cramps (usually the calf), 93% reported an improvement. Such results are overwhelmingly significant.

A Comprehensive Listing of Conditions

The following table contains a comprehensive listing of conditions which have shown to be responsive to antioxidant supplementation in general:

- Attention Deficit Disorder
- AIDS
- Alcoholism
- Allergies
- Anti-aging
- Arthritis
- Asthma
- Atherosclerosis
- Blood circulation

- Blood pressure
- Bronchitis
- Bronchopulmonary Dysplasia
- Bruises
- Bursitis
- Cancer
- Capillary resistance
- Cataracts
- Chelation
- Cholesterol
- Chronic Fatigue Syndrome (CFS)
- Colds
- Cold Sores
- Collagen
- Cramps e.g. leg
- Crohn's Disease
- Depression
- Dermatitis
- Diabetes
- Diabetic retinopathy
- Drug Abuse
- Cirrhosis
- Eczema
- Edema
- Elasticity (blood vessels)
- Fatigue
- Hay fever
- Hemolytic anemia (Anemia)
- Hemorrhage
- Hemorrhoids
- Hyperactivity (ADD)
- Immune enhancer
- Infertility (Male)
- Infection
- Inflammation
- Intestines
- Joint flexibility
- Leg cramps
- Leukemia
- Liver (Cirrhosis)
- Lymph Nodes
- Memory
- Menopause
- Menorrhagia (Heavy Periods)
- Multiple Sclerosis
- Muscle weakness
- Nail problems
- Oral hygiene
- Phlebitis
- PMS
- Prostate
- Psoriasis
- Pulmonary embolism
- Radiation sickness
- Rejuvenates
- Revitalizes (skin)
- Scurvy
- Senility

- Sick Child Syndrome
- Skin eruptions
- Sports injuries
- Stomach ulcer
- Stress
- Stroke
- Sunburn

- Thrombosis
- Trauma
- Tumors
- Ulcers
- Urticaria
- Varicose veins
- Wrinkles

Chapter 9

Pycnogenol Supplementation

THE NOTED medical nutritionist, Lendon Smith, M.D. has commented that he has always, innately, eaten apples and grapes, whole, including the skin and even chewing up the seeds. At one point he rationalized that he must be getting something akin to vitamin A. Now he ponders that his taste buds may have led him to boost his consumption of Pycnogenols!

General Guidelines

Today in America, and over the past two decades in Europe, most people prefer to receive a convenient, concentrated tablet or capsule, usually averaging around 50 mg of Pycnogenol, requiring, typically, between one and six tablets per day. Some consumers calculate their dosage according to body weight (i.e., 1–1.5 mg per pound; or 1 tablet per 50 pounds) with an extra one or two to combat extra stress, or infection; or, indeed, the stresses of infection!.

James D. Krystosik, D.C. conveniently summarized many of Professor Masquelier's suggested dosages from his book, *OPC in Practice.*

The typical standard, or maintenance, dosage that Professor Masquelier recommends is 1.5 mg per 3 pounds of body weight for adults and half that for children on a daily basis.

Someone weighing 180 pounds would require 270 mgs of Pycnogenol™, which would be conveniently rounded up to 300 mg: 4 × 75 mg tablets, or 6 × 50 mg The former might be most easily taken singly with meals and at bedtime; the latter in pairs, at meal times.

In the event of an infection the adult dose increases to 1.5 mg per pound of body weight, i.e. three-fold the regular dose.

This loading or "saturation" level may be maintained for up to three months. Some people take this whole dose at one time, usually at night for a month or two.

Specific Guidelines

Some specific recommendations for common conditions are as follows:

- **Arthritis**—100–150 mg at bed time. Take with marine lipids (fish oils EPA/DHA) and/or shark cartilage.
- **Capillary resistance**—100–150 mg a day. Take with vitamin C.
- **Cholesterol**—Saturate (1.5 mg/pound) for 1 month, then continue with daily maintenance dose (1.5 mgs/ 3 pounds). Take with vitamin C and psyllium seeds (fiber).
- **Diabetic retinopathy**—100–150 mg for the first 10 days then maintain with 40–80 mg per day. Take with bilberry. [Recent research presented by Dr. John M. Ellis highly recommends the use of vitamin B_6 (pyridoxine): 100–300 mg daily, with amelioration taking up to 3 months, followed by a maintenance dose, usually 100 mg]
- **Edema**—150 mg (up to 300 mg in severe conditions) for 1 or 2 months. Continue with maintenance dose.
- **Leg cramps**—150 mg daily for 1 or 2 months followed by maintenance program. Take with vitamin E and minerals: calcium and magnesium.

- **PMS** (Pre-menstrual syndrome)—1.5 mg per pound for 2 to 4 weeks, then a daily maintenance program. Take with B_6 and evening primrose oil.
- **Sports Injuries/Trauma**—150 mg per day for acute inflammation and pain (10 days). Take with homeopathic arnica.
- **Swollen Lymph Nodes**—Loading dose for 1 to 2 months, then daily maintenance.
- **Varicose Veins**—150 mg Daily for 1 to 2 months, then daily maintenance program. Take with vitamin E and cayenne pepper.

Chapter 10

Aromatherapeutic Pine Oil

WITH THE recent renewal of interest in aromatherapy, pine oil (remember Pycnogenol was originally derived from maritime pine) has been recommended for soothing liver problems, among other uses.

Essential oil of pine is obtained from Pinus sylvestris, the Scotch or Norwegian Pine, and it is very important to know the source of the oil, with its botanical name, as there are many species and varieties of Pine with very different properties and uses, and at least one, Dwarf Pine (Pinus pumilo) is classed as a hazardous oil.

The chief uses of Pine are in the treatment of chest infections. Avicenna (980–1037 A.D.) regarded it as a specific for pneumonia and other lung infections It is an expectorant and has a very powerful antiseptic, stimulating effect on circulation. Pine is sometimes used to relieve rheumatic pain.

The essential oil is very pale yellow with a strong, fresh resinous aroma. Its main constituents include acetate of bornyl (up to 45%) cadinene, sylvestrene, dipentene and phellandrene.

It is important to use pure essential pine oil. Positive results have been produced by applying pine oil topically—rubbing in through the skin, 15 drops 1–2 times daily around the liver area, just under the right rib cage, front and back.

The pure essential pine oil when coupled with other antioxidants seems to increase their effect for some unknown reason. Some skin irritations can be corrected by mixing the pine oil with pure essential aloe vera oil. Of course, it is better to discover that one is sensitive to the oil before using it over the whole body! Try a small area along the forearm, for example, as with a perfume sample.

Chapter 11

Safety and Toxicity

PYCNOGENOL, like the other plant-derived antioxidants, has been used for many centuries in its original, natural form, and for decades in the modern extracted version, with no reports of any adverse effects.

The controversial Ames Test has caused quercitin to be labeled "mutagenic," but the validity is disputed, together with similar results for vitamin C itself and rutin. Rutin, like other bioflavonoids, has a low toxicity and is generally recognized as safe.

In particular, Pycnogenol has been subjected to rigorous testing at prestigious centers like the Pasteur Institute in France, a center in Finland and several centers in Germany. Pycnogenol was found to be nontoxic, nonteratogenic, nonmutagenic, noncarcinogenic and nonantigenic—in a word, *safe*.

The manufacturing company, Horphag, conducts routine toxicological tests under the standards of its domestic market, Switzerland—a country renowned for precision.

In the typically reserved style of an academic, Professor Antti H. Arstila responded to a discussion on the safety of Pycnogenol with the leading American researcher on the subject, Dr. Richard Passwater, by saying that Pycnogenol, "is safe as a daily food supplement when used as recommended."

Actually, just as water and oxygen can be toxic at saturation levels, there is a lethal dose for Pycnogenol. In animal studies, the level was 3 gms per kilogram of body weight, almost half a pound for the average adult, equivalent to the supply required for maintenance dosage over a period of five years!

Being water soluble, Pycnogenol must be taken daily, otherwise it is excreted and the protective effect lost.

On a more positive note, Dr. Peter Rohdewald of the Pharmacology Institute of the University of Munster addressed the International Pycnogenol Symposium held in Bordeaux during 1990. In summation, he stated that: "Pycnogenol is a safe, natural product with no adverse effects whatsoever."

Abstracts

A review of the functions of Vitamin C

This is a review of a symposium sponsored by the National Cancer Institute on vitamin C. The symposium was entitled, "Ascorbic Acid: Biological Functions and Relation To Cancer." It was held September 10–12, 1990 at the Lister Hill Auditorium at the National Institute of Health in Bethesda, Maryland. Forty papers were presented and one-hundred thirty scientists and doctors were present from all over the world.

Dr. Balz Frei, from the University of California at Berkeley, shared his work which showed that no cancer causing chemical reaction (ex. lipid peroxidation) could be detected in human plasma as long as vitamin C was present. Lipid peroxidation would return when vitamin C was gone.

Dr. Niki, from the University of Tokyo, stated that free radicals were destroyed faster by vitamin C than by any other antioxidant.

Dr. Linus Pauling noted that many animals manufacture the equivalent per body weight of 10,000 mg/d of vitamin C. He reviewed studies where mice, exposed to carcinogenic ultraviolet light, were given varying amounts of vitamin C, which resulted in reductions and delay in cancerous lesion formation. With increased vitamin C consumption in mice with spontaneous mammary tumors, delayed appearance of these tumors occurred.

Two different researchers from the Linus Pauling Institute for Science and Medicine in Palo Alto, California, Drs. Raxit J. Jariwalla and Constance S. Tsao, reported on the benefits of vitamin C. Dr. Jariwalla showed that vitamin C in AIDS may inhibit a key viral enzyme needed for viral replication; it also reduced extracellular levels of p24 core protein. Dr. Tsao showed that vitamin C, in conjunction with cupric sulfate, had antitumor activity on human mammary tumor fragments implanted in mice.

Dr. Joachim Liehr from the University of Texas at Galveston reported that vitamin C inhibited the incidence of kidney tumors induced by estradiol and diethyl-stilbesterol. Pretreatment of hamsters with vitamin C protected them against the cancer causing effects of DES injections.

In mice models, Dr. Poydock showed complete inhibition of cancer cell growth with a vitamin C and B_{12} combination. Dr. Poydock from the Mercyhurst College Cancer Research Center in Erie, Pennsylvania, who did these studies, gave a case report of a patient with adenocarcinoma of the lung treated intravenously with vitamin C/B_{12} and the tumor was reduced significantly after three treatments.

Dr. Okunieff from the Radiology Department at Harvard Medical School reported that vitamin C given to laboratory animals just prior to radiation therapy showed a significant reduction in skin damage. A similar effect on bone marrow was also seen. In animals, Dr. Okunieff reported vitamin C necessitated only half as much radiation as those without vitamin C at forty-day survival.

Dr. Gary Meadows, from Washington State University, found vitamin C supplementation in the drinking water of mice inhibited cancer growth, enhanced the benefit of chemotherapeutic agents, and in combination or by itself increased survival time of tumor bearing mice.

Dr. Marcus from Lederle Laboratory in Pearl River, New York, found vitamin C usage was increased with high dose interleukin therapy and suggested vitamin C should be used as an adjunctive treatment while utilizing interleukin at high dose.

Dr. Kan Shimpo from the Institute of Comprehensive Medical Sciences, School of Medicine Fujita Health, University of Japan, found vitamin C decreased the toxicity of the cancer drug adriamycin. Vitamin C prevented elevation of lipid peroxides from adriamycin administration.

Dr. Jacob from the USDA Western Nutrition Research Center in San Francisco took eight healthy men and put them on a very low vitamin C diet of 5-20 mg/d for sixty days and found levels of fecal mutagens to be increased significantly.

Dr. Mark Levine from the Laboratory of Cell Biology and Genetics reported on NIDDKD, a technique for assessing optimal vitamin C status, which he calls "in situ kinetics."

Dr. Block from the Division of Cancer Prevention and Control at the National Cancer Institute, ended the symposium with a review of all the studies showing vitamin C having a protective effect in preventing cancer. The sites include the lung, larynx, oral cavity, esophagus, stomach, colon, rectum, pancreas, bladder, cervix, childhood brain tumors, endometrium and breast. Out of forty-seven studies, thirty-four found vitamin C to have a protective effect from cancer at these sites. The amount of vitamin C that may be protective was stated by Dr. Block to be approximately 380 mg/d. Those who had the top 25% of vitamin C intake had one-half the cancer risk from those in the bottom 25% of vitamin C intake.

A report in the *Journal of the National Cancer Institute* ([1990]; 82:561–569) stated: "Vitamin C had the most consistent and statistically significant inverse association with breast cancer risk".... "If all postmenopausal women in the population modify their saturated fat intake to a level of the lower 1/5th of the population, the current rate of breast cancer would be reduced by 10% in North American women. If all postmenopausal women in the population were to increase fruit and vegetable intake to reach an average daily consumption of vitamin C equaling the level among women in the upper 1/5th of the population the risk of breast cancer would be reduced by 16%."

Twenty-two of thirty-two studies showed a cancer protective benefit from increased fruit intake. It was also noted that blacks on the average have a much lower vitamin C serum level than whites, as well as a higher cancer incidence and lower five year cancer survival rate. From these studies it was clear that increased vitamin C intake and fruit consumption are major preventive agents in cancer risk reduction.

The NCI will be evaluating Dr. Pauling and his colleagues' work on thirty cancer patients treated with vitamin C by a panel of twelve specialists in a meeting in December, 1990.

Klein, Morton A. "A Major Symposium on Vitamin C Sponsored by The National Cancer Institute." December 1990, pp. 7. (Address: Linus Pauling Institute of Science and Medicine, 440 Page Mill Road, Palo Alto, CA 94306-2025, USA 415-327-4064)

Exercise, Vitamins and Muscle Loss

Muscle (or lean body mass) is linked with aging. As muscle mass decreases, the elderly have increased problems with mobility and balance, which contributes to the increased risk of falls. It has been shown that highly trained athletes in their 70s have the same muscle mass as 25-year-olds. Free radicals are noted to be related to heart disease, cancer, cataracts, Parkinson's disease, senile macular degeneration and some forms of arthritis and photodermatoses. However, the antioxidant nutrients including vitamins C, E and beta-carotene, protect the body from excess free radicals. Vitamins B_6, B_{12} and folic acid may also be used to decrease some forms of vascular disease.

Degenerative conditions decrease in patients with high-circulating levels, or diets high in these nutrients, according to Dr. Irwin Rosenberg, director of the USDA Human Nutrition Research Center on Aging at Tufts University School of Medicine.

Kubetin, Sally Koch. "Exercise, Vitamins Help Avert Muscle Loss in Elderly." *Family Practice News*. (May 1, 1993); 50.

Role of Vitamins in Reducing Disability and Improving Quality of Life in the Elderly

This report reviews the role of vitamins in reducing disability and improving quality of life in the elderly. Although people over 65 years-of-age comprised 11% of the U.S. population in 1980, they accounted for approximately 29% of personal health expenditure. Various intervention studies of the elderly have included administering antioxidant mixtures containing beta-carotene, vitamins C, E and B complex or multivitamins. A variety of studies have shown antioxidant vitamins with or without selenium and/or other vitamins can improve age-associated memory impairment or various aspects of dementia.

In one study, the Hamilton Depression Scale score was shown to be inversely related with vitamin B_6 plasma levels. Carotene, riboflavin and hematocrit were negatively associated with the Hamilton Depression Scale. The more severe the depression, the lower the vitamin status.

The Mini-Mental Total Score was positively correlated with ascorbic acid plasma levels, suggesting that the higher the cognitive score, the higher the plasma vitamin C. The worse the Activity of Daily Living score, the lower the carotene and riboflavin status. There was also a large number of inverse associations between the Sandoz Clinical Assessment-Geriatric Scale and vitamins B_1, B_2 and C, folic acid and retinol. The author concludes that micronutrients play an important role in the mental state of the elderly. The intervention studies should provide conclusive evidence for the beneficial actions of micronutrients on mental performance and other factors that affect the quality of life of the elderly.

Haller, J. "Vitamins For the Elderly: Reducing Disability and Improving Quality of Life." *Aging Clinical and Experimental Research.* (1993); 5 (Suppl. 1):65–70.

Aging, Atherosclerosis and Cancer

This article extensively reviews the role of free radicals on cancer and atherosclerosis. Aerobic creatures are not only dependent on oxygen, but are exposed to it; though humans may be exposed to more oxidant stress. There is indirect evidence implicating reactive oxygen species in diseases such as cancer and atherosclerosis. Oxidative stress may be a normal process of aging. Oxidative stress can be measured by such techniques as breath pentane, electronic spin resonance and specific measures of base damage to DNA by mass spectrometry and other techniques. Important data will be revealed soon from large scale chemoprevention trials currently underway. Free radical scavenging enzymes can be assessed and can compliment the more routine measurements of trace elements and antioxidant nutrients.

Bankson, Daniel, D. et al., "Role of Free Radicals in Cancer and Atherosclerosis." *Clinics in Laboratory Medicine*, (1993); 13(2):463–480.

The Prevention of Atherosclerosis With Antioxidants

This is a review article on the role of antioxidants in atherosclerosis. The antioxidant drug probucol has a hypocholesterolemic and antioxidant effect, which helps prevent oxidation of LDL cholesterol. It is also noted that research has shown that vitamins C and E, beta-carotene, and monounsaturated fatty acids, when they replace polyunsaturated fatty acids, can reduce the susceptibility to LDL oxidation. In the future, antioxidant therapy, in conjunction with lipid lowering regimes, may play a key role in the prevention of atherosclerosis.

Harris, William S., Ph.D. "The Prevention of Atherosclerosis With Antioxidants." *Clinical Cardiology*. (1992); 15:636–640.

Acquired Atherosclerosis: Theories of Causation, Novel Therapies

This article states that there are eight theories which try to explain atherosclerosis: A. Cholesterol, B. Homocysteine, C. Antioxidant, D. Viral damage, E. Free-radical, F. LDL-modification, G. Clonal, and H. Micronutrient hypotheses. The author states that each hypothesis has some truth to it. This article reviews the concept that atherosclerosis is a vitamin deficiency disease. One main premise is that the western diet is high in protein and low in vitamin B_6. This can increase the risk to oxysterols which can result in arterial damage as well as damage to LDL cholesterol. The author also notes that vitamin B_6 is very important in the metabolism of homocysteine. Low B_6 levels result in elevated homocysteine which can lead to oxidant stress in atherosclerosis. Reduction of these oxysterols can occur from reduced amounts of refined foods, especially oils, as well as the consumption of other antioxidants including vitamin E 100 to 200 I.U., vitamin C 2 to 4 gms, selenium 100 mcgs, and Coenzyme Q 10 between 10 and 30 mgs per day. The author compares cultures which have low incidences or high incidences of heart disease, and correlates that with high or low levels of vitamin B_6. In conclusion, the dietary factors that increase the risk to atherosclerosis include high protein diets and the consumption of processed, prepackaged foods which may contain high amounts of oxysterols.

Hattersley, Joseph G. "Acquired Atherosclerosis: Theories of Causation, Novel Therapies." *Journal of Orthomolecular Medicine.* (1991);6(2):83–98.

Antioxidants and Polyunsaturated Fatty Acids

Ninety-one patients with varying degrees of coronary artery disease were compared to seventy-two controls for the degree of atherosclerosis and its relationship to selenium, alpha tocopherol (vitamin E) and serum polyunsaturated fatty acid levels. Plasma selenium was significantly lower in patients than in controls. The ratio of selenium to linoleic acid, selenium to total polyunsaturated fatty acids and selenium to total omega-6 fatty acids was significantly lower in coronary artery disease patients. These relationships were more significant in individuals with low vitamin E levels. The authors hypothesize that high polyunsaturated fatty acids with insufficient antioxidant protection may increase the risk of cardiovascular disease.

Kok, Frans, J. et al., "Do Antioxidants and Polyunsaturated Fatty Acids Have a Combined Association With Coronary Atherosclerosis." *Arteriosclerosis.* (1991);31:85–90.

Antioxidant Properties of bioflavonoids

A pro-oxidant drug, primaquine (PQ) was used to produce oxidative stress in human red blood cells (RBC) in vitro. Rutin, a plant flavonoid, did not prevent PQ-induced cell lysis but protected against hemoglobin (Hb) oxidation inside RBC. The present results demonstrate new antioxidant properties of rutin that may be useful in diminishing oxidative damage to pathological red blood cells.

Grinberg, L.N., E.A. Rachmilewitz, and H. Newmark. "Protective Effects of Rutin Against Hemoglobin Oxidation." *Biochem-Pharmacol.* (1994); 17; 48(4): 643–9.

Free Radical Scavenging and Antioxidative Effects of Flavonoids.

The abilities of fifteen flavonoids as scavengers of active oxygens (hydroxyl radical and superoxide anion) were studied. Hydroxyl radical (.OH) was generated by the Fenton system, and assayed by the determination of methanesulfonic acid (MSA) formed from the reaction of dimethyl sulfoxide

(DMSO) with .OH. (+)-Catechin, (-)-epicatechin, 7,8-dihydroxy flavone, and rutin showed the .OH scavenging effect 100–300 times superior to that of mannitol, a typical .OH scavenger.

Hanasaki, Y., S. Ogawa, and S. Fukui. "The Correlation Between Active Oxygens Scavenging and Antioxidative Effects of Flavonoids." *Free-Radic-Biol-Med.* (1994); 16(6): 845–50.

Effects of GLA, Flavonoids & Vitamins on Lipid Peroxidation.

Gamma linolenic acid (GLA), a polyunsaturated fatty acid, promoted lipid peroxidation. The increase could be correlated with cytotoxicity. The plant flavonoids (quercetin, luteolin, butein, rutin) and the fat-soluble components (retinol, retinoic acid, alpha-tocopherol) by themselves did not affect lipid peroxidation. Quercetin, luteolin, retinol, and alpha-tocopherol were able to inhibit cell proliferation significantly.

Interestingly, the cytotoxic actions of these well-known natural antioxidants do not involve free radicals or lipid peroxidation reactions.

Ramanathan, R. et al. "Effects of Gamma-Linolenic Acid, Flavonoids, and Vitamins on Cytotoxicity and Lipid Peroxidation." *Free-Radic-Biol-Med.* (Jan 1994); 16(1): 43–8.

References:

Blazso, G., and M. Gabor. "Influence of O-(beta-hydroxyethyl)-Rutin on the Edema-Inhibiting Effect of Indomethacin." *Acta-Pharm-Hung* (July 1994); 64(4): 123–4.

Carlotti, M.E., M. Gallarate, M.R. Gasco, and M. Trotta. "Inhibition of Lipoperoxidation of Linoleic Acid by Five Antioxidants of Different Lipophilicity." *Pharmazie.* (Jan 1994); 49(1): 49–52.

Cody, V. et al. "Plant Flavonoids in Biology and Medicine: Biochemical, Cellular and Medicinal Properties." *New York, Liss.* 1988.

Cureton, T.K. *Medicina Deportiva.* (1958) 12: 259–263.

Elangovan, V., N. Sekar, and S. Govindasamy. "Chemopreventive Potential of Dietary Bioflavonoids Against 20-methylcholanthrene Induced Tumorigenesis." *Cancer-Lett.* (Nov 25, 1994); 87(1): 107–13.

Elstner, E.F. and E. Kleber. "Flavoinoids in Biology and Medicine." *Current Issues In Flavonoids Research.* (1990) National University of Singapore, pp. 227–235.

Grinberg, L. N., E.A. Rachmilewitz, and H. Newmark. "Protective Effects of Rutin Against Hemoglobin Oxidation." *Biochem-Pharmacol.* (Aug 17, 1994); 48(4): 643–9.

Hanasaki, Y., S. Ogawa, and S. Fukui. "The Correlation Between Active Oxygens Scavenging and Antioxidative Effects of Flavonoids." *Free-Radic-Biol-Med.* (June 1994); 16(6): 845–50.

Harborne, J.B. *The Flavonoids: Advances in Research Since 1980.* London, Chapman & Hall, 1988.

Hendrickson, H.P., A.D. Kaufman, and C.E. Lunte. "Electrochemistry of Catechol-Containing Flavonoids." *J-Pharm-Biomed-Anal.* (Mar 1994); 12(3): 325–34.

Kootstra, A. "Protection from UV-B-Induced DNA Damage by Flavonoids." *Plant-Mol-Biol.* (Oct 1994); 26(2): 771–4.

Krystosik, James, D. *Pycnogenol—Nature's Prescription for Aging, Allergies...* Garrettsville, OH: Good News Press, 1995.

Laparra, J., J. Michaud, and G. Masquelier. *Plantes Médicinales et Phytothérapie.* (1978); 4:233.

Laparra, J., J. Michaud, M.F. Lesca, P. Blanquet, and G. Masquelier. *Acto Therapeutica,* (1978); 4:233.

Larocca, L.M., M. Giustacchini, N. Maggiano, F.O. Ranelletti, M. Piantelli, E. Alcini, and A. Capelli. "Growth-Inhibitory Effect of Quercetin and Presence of Type II Estrogen Binding Sites in Primary Human Transitional Cell Carcinomas." *J. Urol.* (Sep 1994); 152(3); 1029–33.

Mahady, G.B., and C.W. Beecher. "Quercetin-Induced Benzophenanthridine Alkaloid Production in Suspension Cell Cultures of Sanguinaria Canadensis." *Planta-Med.* (Dec 1994); 60(6): 553–7.

Masquelier, J., J. Michaud, J. Laparra, and M.C. Dumon. *Intern. J. Vit. Nutr. Res,* (1979); 49:307.

Masquelier, J., J. Michaud, J. Laparra, and M.C. Dumon. *Bull Soc Pharm.* Bordeaux (1979); 118:95

Micozzi, Marc S. "Plant Flavonoids—Can They Heal Us?" *Executive Health's Good Health Report.* January 1993, 29(4):1–4.

Middleton, E., and C. Kandaswami. *The Flavonoids: Advances in Research Since 1986.* London: Chapman & Hall, 1993.

Murray, Michael T., "PCO Sources: Grape Seed Vs Pine Bark—A Review and Comparison." *Health Counselor.* Vol 7(1), provided as a brochure by Enzymatic Therapy of Green Bay, Wisconsin.

Oyama, Y., P.A. Fuchs, N. Katayama, and K. Noda. "Myricetin and Quercetin, The Flavonoid Constituents of Ginkgo Biloba Extract, Greatly Reduce Oxidative Metabolism in Both Resting and Ca(2+)-Loaded Brain Neurons." *Brain-Res.* (Jan 28 1994); 635(1-2): 125–9.

Passwater, Richard A., *The New Superoxidant—Plus—The Amazing Story of Pycnogenol™, Free Radical Antagonist and Vitamin Potentiator.* New Canaan, CT: Keats, 1992.

Passwater, Richard A. *Pycnogenol: The Super "Protector" Nutrient.* New Canaan, CT: Keats, 1994.

Peaston, M.J.T., and P. Finnegan. "A Case of Combined Poisoning With Chlorpropamide, Acetylsalicylic Acid and Paracetamol." *British Journal of Clinical Practice.* (1968) 22.

Perez-Guerrero, C., M.J. Martin, and E. Marhuenda. "Prevention by Rutin of Gastric Lesions Induced by Ethanol in Rats: Role of Endogenous Prostaglandins." *Gen-Pharmacol.* (May 1994); 25(3): 575–80.

Ramanathan, R., N.P. Das, and C.H. Tan. "Effects of Gamma-Linolenic Acid, Flavonoids, and Vitamins on Cytotoxicity and Lipid Peroxidation." *Free-Radic-Biol-Med.* (Jan 1994); 16(1): 43–8.

Scambia, G., et-al. "Quercetin Potentiates the Effect of Adriamycin in a Multidrug-Resistant MCF-7 Human Breast-Cancer Cell Line: P-Glycoprotein as a Possible Target." *Cancer-Chemother-Pharmacol.* (1994); 34(6): 459–64.

Thomas, C.L. *Taber's Cyclopedic Medical Dictionary.* Philadelphia: F.A. Davis Co., 1985.

Walji, Hasnain. *The Vitamin Guide—Essential Nutrients for Healthy Living,* Dorset, U.K.: Element Books, 1992.

Walji, Hasnain. *Asthma and Hayfever—Combining Orthodox and Complementary Approaches.* London: Hodder Headline Plc, 1993.

Walji, Hasnain. *Alcohol, Smoking and Tranquillisers.* London: Hodder Headline Plc., 1993.

Walji, Hasnain. *Heart Health. A Self-help Guide to combining Orthodox and Complementary Approaches.* London: Hodder Headline Plc., 1994.

Walji, Hasnain. *Arthritis and Rheumatism—Orthodox and Complementary Approaches.* London: Hodder Headline Plc., 1994.

Walji, Hasnain. *Vitamins, Minerals and Dietary Supplements—A definitive Guide to Healthy Eating.* London: Hodder Headline Plc., 1994.

Walji, Hasnain. *Melatonin.* London: Thorsons-Harper Collins, 1995.

Weiner, Michael, and A. Janet Weiner. *Weiner's Herbal The Guide to Herb Medicine.* New York: Stein and Day, 1980.

Yonei, S., A. Noda, S. Tachibana, and S. Akasaka. *Mutation Res.* (1986) 193:15.

Author Profile

Hasnain Walji, Ph.D., is an expert consultant on natural health and a researcher and writer specializing in nutrition and complementary therapies.

He is the author of *The Vitamin Guide—Essential Nutrients for Healthy Living*, published by Element Books, and has written six books as part of a new series exploring common ailments from complementary and orthodox points of view published by Hodder Headline Plc. and endorsed by the Natural Medicine Society of England. The titles are: *Asthma and Hayfever, Skin Problems, Addiction, Headaches & Migraine, Arthritis & Rheumatism* and *Heart Health*. The series has been translated into Spanish. Other tiles include *Vitamins, Minerals and Dietary Supplements—A definitive Guide to Healthy Eating* published by Hodder Headline. *Using Aromatherapy at home* published by C.P.R. Publishing, Cleveland, UK

Hasnain has also written a series of books for Thorsons–Harper Collins for their Nutrients for Health Series. The titles include *Melatonin, Vitamin C, Bee Products* and *Folic Acid.*

A contributor to several journals on environmental and Third World consumer issues, he was the founder and editor of *The Vitamin Connection*—an International Journal of Nutrition, Health and Fitness, published in the UK, Canada and Australia, focusing on the link between health and diet. He also launched *Healthy Eating*, a consumer magazine focusing on the concept of optimum nutrition and has written a script for a six part television series, *The World of Vitamins*, to be produced by a Danish Television company

He is also Program Director of Software Development Innovations Inc. (Dallas, Texas) the publishers and developers of The Natural Health Information System™ which comprises of an interactive suite of Programs called NutriPlus™ and Health Plus™. He lives in Milton Keynes and spends his time between UK and USA.

Index

swollen lymph nodes   68
varicose veins   68

H

hay fever   25, 49, 64
hemolytic anemia (Anemia)   64
hemorrhage   64
hemorrhoids   64
hyperactivity (ADD)   64
hepatitis   35
herpes   35
HIV   47

I

immune system   14–15, 17–23, 25, 27–29, 34, 35, 42, 44, 47, 50–51, 59, 61, 64
  enhancer   64
  free radicals   22
  thymus gland   18
  zinc   29
immunoglobulins
    See antibodies
infection   64
infertility (male)   64
inflammation   64
intestines   64

J

joint flexibility   64
joint trauma   38

K

Krystosik, James D., D.C.
   46, 57, 66

L

leg cramps   64, 67
leukemia   64
Levine, Dr. Mark   28
Lind, James   4
liver (cirrhosis)   64
lymph nodes   64

M

macronutrients   24
male infertility   64
malnutrition   14
Masquelier, Jacques   5
measles   35
medication   42
  vitamin C   42
Melatonin   2, 23
memory   64
menopause   64
menorrhagia (heavy periods)   64
Micozzi, Dr. Marc S.   9
micronutrients   24
Multiple Sclerosis   64
Muscle weakness (loss)   64, 76

N

nail problems   64
National Institute of Health   28

O

oral hygiene   64
Oxygen
  free radicals   21

P

R

S

sunburn 65
swollen lymph nodes 68

T

T-cells 16, 17, 34
thrombosis 65
thymus gland
  immunity 19
  lymphocytes 18
trauma 65
tumors 65, 73

U

ulcers 65
urticaria 65

V

Varicose Veins 36, 63, 65,
  68
vitamin A 26, 27, 33
  antioxidant 26
  skin cancer 58
vitamin B_6 27
vitamin B_{12} 27
vitamin C 1–5, 8, 10, 11–
  12, 23, 26, 28–29, 32–
  42, 47, 50–53, 56–57, 60,
  62, 67, 71, 73–75,77, 79

alcohol 41
antibiotics 42
antioxidant 28
arthritis 50
burns 51
cancer 51
cataracts 53
energy 62
functions of 73
illness 35
RDA 36, 39
skin cancer 58
stress 62
vitamin E
  11, 23, 29, 33, 36, 58
  antioxidant 29
  atherosclerosis 80
  skin cancer 58
vitamin P 1, 10
  bioflavonoid 4

W

White, Dr. David 55
wounds 38
wrinkles 65

Z

zinc 23, 29, 36
  antioxidant 29